Promise and Peril

The last five years have been a time of promise and peril in biomedical research. Genetic engineering has made plentiful such once-rare drugs as interferon, growth hormone, and human insulin. After years of work, an experimental artificial heart entered human testing. Slowly, scientists have begun to unlock the mysteries of cancer's origins. In these and many other developments, research has lengthened and enriched our lives.

Yet for each new life-saving technology, each advance in the control of life processes, we face new ethical problems.

Explore these developments, the people behind the formal mask of science, the very human process of discovery—all in THE OMNI BOOK OF MEDICINE. . . .

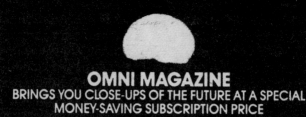

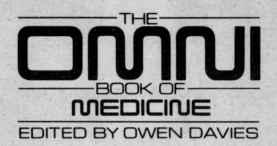

THE OMNI
BOOK OF
MEDICINE

EDITED BY OWEN DAVIES

ZEBRA BOOKS
KENSINGTON PUBLISHING CORP.

THE OMNI
BOOK OF
MEDICINE

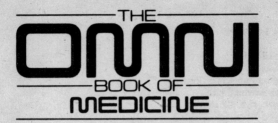

CONTENTS

PART THREE: HEALING

PART FOUR: HERITAGE

PART FIVE: MIND

PART SIX: OF SCIENCE BORN

PART SEVEN: PATHWAYS
TOWARD PROGRESS

PART EIGHT: BIOETHICS

FOREWORD

In the world of science, few disciplines are as fast-moving as biomedical research. Few are as able to touch our lives. Few are as heavily publicized. And yet few are less well known.

Each morning in the newspaper, each night on television, we hear of discovery. New drugs and vaccines, new insights into the workings of life have appeared almost routinely since James Watson and Francis Crick worked out the structure of DNA some thirty years ago. Yet what we read and hear is just the surface, results arrived at by years of patient research that television hasn't the time to explain.

For every headline, hundreds of experiments go unnoticed except by the few scientists whose work they advance. It is among these little-known studies that we can find the future. Searching it out is the special role of *Omni* magazine.

When *Omni* first appeared, in October 1978, it set a new standard for science journalism. *Omni* writers understood both science and scientists. They could report a finding as well as the best newsmen, but they could also explain how it came about and where it would lead. They could reveal the people behind the formal mask of science and bring alive the very human process of discovery. Best of all, they could *write*. They could write about the world of science as vividly as Red Smith could recreate a pennant-winning catch. Heady stuff in a field where second-string newsmen were used to touting every new diet and baldness remedy as a medical breakthrough.

Omni's five years have been a time of promise and peril in biomedical research. Genetic engineering has made plentiful such once-rare drugs as interferon, growth hormone, and human insulin. After years of work, an experimental artificial heart entered human testing. Slowly, scientists have begun to unlock the mysteries of cancer's origins. In these and many other developments, research has lengthened and enriched our lives.

Yet for each new life-saving technology, each advance in the control of life processes, we face new ethical problems. Can we fix genetic ills without being tempted to mold future generations to our own liking? Does the unborn right to life void the unwilling mother's right to an abortion? Should doctors withhold "heroic" treatments for the hopelessly ill? These and many other medical issues have grown ever more difficult.

In covering all these developments, *Omni* has led the field from the first. In the magazine's first issue, staff writer Kathleen Stein explored research into the processes of aging. "Some of Us

May Never Die," she called her article; she was right. The next month found free-lance writer Dick Teresi, now *Omni*'s editor, visiting the University of Utah for a look at the work on artificial organs; this was four years before Seattle dentist Barney Clark and his mechanical heart carried the Utah program into the headlines. And a few months later, scientists Sandy Shaw and Durk Pearson contributed their first article for laymen: "Mind Food," a menu of nutrients and drugs that may strengthen the memory and sharpen the intellect. It would be three years before their book, "Life Extension" reached the best-seller lists.

These and many of the articles that have followed them are gathered into this volume. Individually, they give entertaining, indepth stories from the frontiers of biomedical research. As a group, they provide a rare look at the future and at the longer, healthier lives we will live in it. In all of them, you will find not just the facts but the people who made them, not just reporting but energy and style that other science magazines can only envy.

— Owen Davies

PART ONE:
AN END TO AGING

SOME OF US MAY NEVER DIE

by Kathleen Stein

In October, 1976, Luna, the 16-year-old daughter of science writer Robert Anton Wilson, was brutally beaten and killed in a grocery store robbery. Helpless in the face of death, Wilson took the only action he could. He had the child's brain set immediately in cryonic suspension, frozen in liquid nitrogen at 320 degrees below zero (Fahrenheit). From this brain a part of Luna's identity may someday be reconstructed, or, from one of her stem cells, a new body cloned. Hers was the first brain to be frozen in this manner. Now, however, a special cryonic cylinder for the brain has been made available for the purpose of future cloning or identity reconstruction of some other kind.

Cryonic preservation is undertaken on the premise that the infinitely more advanced medical scientists of the future might be able to revive the dead and repair whatever killed them. It's a long shot, to say the least, but the odds are still better with freezing than they are with cremation or burial. Some cryobiologists estimate that certain bodies could be preserved for several hundred thousand years without any deterioration.

However desperate, bizarre, or macabre an effort it may seem, cryobiological interest is growing and profit-making organizations such as Trans Time in Berkeley, Bay Area Cryonics, and the Cryonics Society of Michigan are forming around the country. Adherents of the practice include people such as Woody Allen and Columbia University physicist Gerald Feinberg, who conceived the hypothetical faster-than-light particle, the tachyon. It is rumored, although without confirmation, that Walt Disney is among those whose animation is cooling off until a better day.

Unlike Luna Wilson's body, most of the souls resting in cryonic suspension are intact. Immediately after death each body is packed in dry ice, drained of blood and filled with glycerol and DMSO (dimethyl-sulfoxide) an antifreezing agent, to prevent ice crystals from forming in the living tissue. The frozen body is then wrapped in aluminum foil and stored in a thermos-like insulated double-walled polished steel "cryonic storage capsule" until the millennium. The body is "buried" in a cryonic cemetery which uses auxiliary power sources to keep it frozen even in the event of a power shortage.

To keep the immortal fire burning, however, is no minor financial undertaking. For most people, the initial cost of interment amounts to about $15,000 with a maintenance charge of

$1800 a year. At Bay Area Cryonics a $50,000 insurance policy is said to cover the whole thing. And you have to plan ahead!

DEATH VS. THE PEOPLE

The obvious drawback to cryonic suspension is that you have to die in order to enjoy an extended life. But movements such as cryobiology point to the growing rebelliion against aging and death. People simply want to live longer, better, and are less and less willing to "go gentle into that good night." And the cryonic refrigeration revolution with its "freeze . . . wait . . . reanimate" is not the only front on which death and aging are being attacked.

In Robert Anton Wilson's *Cosmic Trigger*, Paul Segall, Ph.D., a researcher in the department of physiology at the University of California, Berkeley, offers several approaches to longevity, which include:

• *Transplantation*, which might allow us to continue replacing organs "until the point where 'we' are still there, but our entire bodies are new."

• *Prosthetics* and *cyborgs*, machine-human combinations of which the Bionic Woman is a none-too-fanciful projection.

• *Identity reconstruction* through cloning.

• *Regeneration*, a process by which repressed genes are switched back on to renew cell tissue.

And at the heart of the matter is *gerontology*. This science investigates not only the chemical and biological processes of aging, but also the possibilities for extended healthy life. If gerontology research proves as promising as it looks, drastic measures such as freezing, cloning, and mechanizing humans in order to preserve your vital personality may not be necessary. Most efforts in the gerontological field are concerned with postponing senescence.

As early as 1962, Dr. Bernard Strehler, professor of biology at the University of Southern California, and one of the indefatigable warriors of the seige on death, announced that before long science will have understood aging's sources and that "toothless, wrinkled, mindless incontinent wrecks with Dorian Gray-like [sic] bodies — they will not exist!" In the absence of aging, Strehler said, the longevity of a healthy 21 year old could exceed 2000 years.

Following the startling hypothesis that aging could be curable, gerontologists have been piecing the puzzle together, moving closer to pinpointing the causes of aging, the sources of longevity.

Right now it seems quite possible that the underlying cause of aging may not be impossibly complex, but singular, primary. It may be that senescence is not a natural phenomenon, but a by-product of social conditions. There may be, in fact, no biological limit to a healthy vigorous lifespan. To extend the accepted lifespan potential from 70— 100 years to 120, 200, 400, 1000 and on up, may be part of *Homo sapiens* on-going evolutionary destiny.

With the tremendous explosion of knowledge of basic molecular biology and genetics, we are learning the secrets of life and in doing so, we're learning how to control aging, to extend life.

Data now are beginning to indicate that life-extension is inevitable. We may have some way of lengthening our lives before the year 2000. Some of us may never die.

An array of potentially useful drugs are in various stages of testing, drugs which may not extend lifespan significantly, but which will stave off bodily wear and tear, perhaps rejuvenate the body and preserve energy and youthfulness past middle age. These drugs might contribute to a "synergistic effect" whereby one advance buys a person enough time to live well until the subsequent discovery prolongs his health even more.

Anti-aging therapies are being tested that combat free radicals, for example, those fragments of molecules which break off, career about the body tissue wreaking havoc and contributing to the build-up of cellular garbage such as lipofuscins. Dr. Denham Harman, an internist-chemist at the University of Nebraska school of medicine is working on a series of antioxidants, which react with free radicals and minimize their effects.

Dr. Harman developed a number of compounds that increase life expectancy as much as 50 percent in mice. These include: Vitamin E; 2-MEA (mercaptoethylemine), a compound first used for radiation protection; BHT and Santoquin, commonly used as food preservatives; as well as sodium hypophosphite, an old drug used for the treatment of tuberculosis around 1900. These drugs all have extended life expectancy in mice, and Harman hopes this testing will now extend to larger mammals.

Another compound, DMAE (dimethylaminoethanol), is showing promising results, reports Albert Rosenfeld in his important book, *Pro-Longevity*. DMAE is a lysosome membrane stabilizer, and as such it strengthens cells against damage caused by lipofuscin accumulations. When lysosome membranes are damaged, harmful substances leak out and may be responsible for aging symptoms.

Dr. Richard Hochschild of the Microwave Instrument Company of Del Mar, California, found that by adding DMAE to the water of mice he increased their lifespans significantly. Other investigators have successfully employed centrophenoxine, a synthetic compound derived in part from DMAE, to delay lipofuscin build-up in the brain of guinea pigs. Centrophenoxine, which has almost no toxic side effects, is already used experimentally with apparent success in France to improve the mental abilities of senile patients.

The first drug likely to pass through the FDA's interminable bureaucratic maze, however, is the well-publicized Gerovital, developed in 1945 by Dr. Ana Aslan of the Bucharest Geriatric Institute. In Romania it is possible to get "youth shots" of Gerovital's 2 percent procaine hydrochloride and haematoporphyrin solution from government doctors.

Over the last 25 years, Dr. Aslan has claimed to have cured people of everything from heart disease and arthritis to impotence and gray hair. But few scientists are prepared to sing the drug's praises. Says Dr. Ruth Weg, of Andrus Gerontology Center of the University of Southern California: "We just don't know."

The list of potentially effective drugs, then, is growing geometrically, and the catalogue of agents that offer some chance of alleviating or postponing some debilitating symptoms are imminently testable. In the future, moreover, enzyme cocktails and genetic manipulation in pill form might be as commonplace as valium and birth control pills.

EAT LESS, LIVE LONGER

Since the 1930's, classic laboratory studies show that restricting an animal's diet in the first half of its life can double its lifespan—to the point where a 1000-day old rat can be compared to a 90-year-old human with the body of John Travolta. These experiments have been conducted on everything from one-celled *Tokophrya*, to rotifers, worms, insects, mice, hamsters, and rats with similar results. This is a key concept in the theory of life-extension. Restricting diet delays maturity and increases longevity.

Dr. Roy Walford, a pathologist at the UCLA school of medicine, a man with a reputation among his colleagues for meticulous research, recently has extended this nutritional study to include the testing of mental function. He will find out whether dietary restriction produces long-lived idiots or long-lived supermice. "It may well be the supermice," he says.

In a new development, Walford and his associate Dr. Richard Weindruck have discovered that when dietary restriction is begun in mid-life mice, the animals' immune system seem to be rejuvenated. A chief researcher in immunological systems, and the author of the *The Immunologic Theory of Aging*, Walford has found that in aging not only do the immune cells lose their ability to fight off the body's enemies, but they actually go berserk and turn against the very tissue they are supposed to protect. There is increasing evidence that this autoimmune response is a fundamental symptom of aging, which involves certain self-destructive acts: "like an art performance," Walford laughs.

Two years ago, Walford traveled extensively throughout India to measure body temperature regulation among the yogis. He found that through their yogic practices some could lower their body temperature one-half to one-degree Centigrade.

Why lower body temperature? Walford and others have found that reducing body temperature of humans a few degrees could greatly extend lifespan. "A very minor reduction, about three degrees Fahrenheit," says Bernard Strehler, "could well add as much as 30 years to human life."

Neither Walford nor anyone else, however, has succeeded in lowering temperature in "warm-blooded" (homeothermic) animals, although Walford has experiments with the diverse substances, including marijuana, to determine to what extent they could do the job. Marijuana is the best substance for lowering body temperature, he says. Yet his mice developed a tolerance to the drug, and, after a few weeks of injections it had no effect on their temperatures. "There might be an analogue or chemically similar substitute that could do it," he speculates.

Richard Cutler of the National Institute of Aging's Gerontology Research Center offers the bizarre, but workable, scheme of actually inserting a tiny ceramic device into the blood vessel preceding the hypothalamus (where temperature is controlled). A microwave unit also might be placed in the bedroom. At night during sleep, when the body's metabolic rate is slower, the microwave unit would beam on and the embedded device would, in turn, trick the hypothalamus into thinking the body was in a fever of one or two degrees. The hypothalamus consequently would lower the temperature a degree or so. In the early morning, before awaking, the microwave unit would switch off and the body temperature would be restored to 98.6°F. The user would not be bothered, but might live twice as long.

DEATH CLOCK?

As more is known about the genetic structure of life, biologists are coming to the conclusion that aging is not the result of slow "trashing" of all parts, but may be the result of a genetic program, coded along with the other instructions for the functioning of the cells in its DNA. The big question remains: Are we programmed to die? Is there a "death clock" that turns off the genes one by one? Or is nature simply indifferent to our fate after we've played our part in perpetuating the species? Or does the program for growth and sexual maturity contain within it what Dr. Richard Cutler of the National Institute on Aging calls "pleiotropic processes"—necessary functions which have by-products which in the long run are harmful to your health?

Many investigators on the case are now "pro-clock." Opinions vary drastically and vehemently, however, as to where the time-piece is located. One group theorizes that the aging mechanism occurs at the cellular level. Molecular biologist Dr. Leonard Hayflick discovered evidence that there are only so many times ($\pm$ 50) a cell can divide *in vitro* before its descendants age and die. Thus, Hayflick concluded, the cell has a built-in genetic limit. And ever since the revolutionary "Hayflick Limit" was announced, it has been the target of continuous speculation. Critics scour the territory for evidence to refute it.

Dr. V. J. Cristofalo of Philadelphia's Wistar Institute, for instance, has prolonged cellular life by adding the hormones cortisone and hydrocortisone to culture solutions, thus suggesting that it is hormonal balance that signals the termination of cell division, not tiny clocks.

Dr. David Harrison of Jackson Laboratory, Bar Harbor, Maine, believes certain cells may indeed be immortal (as they were thought to be prior to Hayflick's results). When he transplanted stem cells, which have a large prolificacy capacity, from old animals into young, the old cells functioned as well as the young cells did when both were transplanted into young recipients.

Walford's rejuvenation of middle-aged mice's immunological response, as well as work he had done with congenic mice strains, leads him to believe that control of the entire immune system is located within a small region of genetic material—corresponding to the sixth chromosome in humans. He suspects that this control center is fundamentally involved in the aging process as a whole—that it may be "the man pulling the strings behind the scenes." These strings may involve only a few genes.

THE BRAIN, HORMONES & DECO

Many other scientists now think the program for aging is encoded in the hypothalamus-pituitary system. The hypothalamus, that tiny pea-sized node at the base of the brain, is the master regulator of hormone distribution, and, along with the pituitary and endocrine system, it comprises the regulation network affecting virtually all homeostatic systems as well as growth and sexual development.

The body flashes an uninterrupted series of response and feedback signals between the individual glands and the brain. Aging may disrupt the hypothalamus's ability to run the show. Years of evidence more than suggests that the hypothalamic control of hormonal release goes haywire with aging.

By stimulating the hypothalamus of aged female rats with electric impulses, Dr. Joseph Meites of Michigan State, has successfully reactivated their estrus cycles—put them back in heat. He also has reactivated the ovarian cycles of the old females by feeding them L-Dopa (a dopamine stimulator also used in the treatment of Parkinson's disease), and hormones such as progesterone, epinephrine, and iproniazid.

The exciting thing about this evidence is that the old ovaries still work and can be started up again when the "clock" in the hypothalamus is turned back. The implications for women past the menopause are astounding.

Dr. W. Donner Denckla, Associate Professor of Medicine at Harvard's Thorndike Laboratories, thinks he's close enough to hear the death clock ticking. An intense youngish man with collegiate horn rims and a wry sense of humor, Denckla explained recently to the large audience at a life-extension conference in St. Paul sponsored by the University of Minnesota, that he has "one very strong candidate for the demise of mammals."

Denckla's rather spectacular theory is based on the idea that humans have a built-in mechanism, not for aging, but for death itself. He believes the process of dying is built into our childhood; it starts around age ten.

Denckla proposes that at puberty the pituitary starts releasing an exceedingly powerful hormone, which he calls by the artful acronym DECO (for decreasing O_2 consumption). "This lovely little molecule," he says, "wanders out and progressively throws a block between the body's cells and its circulating thyroxin," the thyroid hormone vital to normal metabolism. Death comes as it does to the Pacific Salmon—by flooding the body with the "death hormone"—only more slowly; so insidiously as to seem not the cause.

In his super-realistic laboratories, Denckla removes the pituitaries (from whence, presumably, issues the DECO) of older rats. And, after adding hormone supplements to their diets, in a matter of months the old animals regain much of their pubescent glory.

One big hitch in the Denckla plan is that, although the pituitary-less rats are rejuvenated to adolescent physiological status, their lifespan does not seem to be prolonged. They die on schedule. It is possible, then, that DECO may serve an important life function.

THE LONGEVITY CLOCK

Richard Cutler is a man with a big plan, which, if it does not embrace all of the manifold theories of aging, is at least compatible with most of them. Cutler is looking, not so much for the causes of aging, as for reasons for the evolution of longevity. There is no genetic program for death, he thinks, but an open-ended potential for unlimited lifespan.

In charge of the Program on Comparative Biochemistry of Mammalian Aging, Cutler constructs his architectonic ideas from sources as eclectic as his background. Cutler personally evolved from a Colorado farmboy into a helicopter designer to a copter company owner at age 18. He discovered college a few years later and proceeded to get degrees in aeronautical and electrical engineering, in physics, and biophysics.

According to Cutler, the rate of aging might very well be regulated by relatively few genes, which we can discover and eventually control. He has reached this conclusion after carefully studying the evolution of long lifespan in humans. It seems that our lifespan increased so rapidly compared to our apelike ancestors that no more than a few genes could have changed during such a brief evolutionary period. Hence, Cutler concludes that only a few genes may control the rate of aging.

Slowing down the aging process doesn't have to be a formidable task. We already know much about what genetic controls are involved. The deceleration is likely to be achieved first by biochemical manipulation of the neuroendocrine system via the hypothalamus-pituitary controls and, later, when more is known, by genetic engineering. "The 'scenario', as they say," remarked Cutler, "is that you'd take a child when he's young, administer hormones to slow down his development and give him an analogue in his food to stimulate anti-aging processes." A person might become sexually mature by 28, full grown at 45, and middle aged by 120.

"I think within ten years, depending on how much we concentrate on learning to manipulate the controls of development, the slowdown might be accomplished," he predicts.

A trickier problem than slowing growth is maintaining the body's level of intrinsic wear and tear fighters, what Cutler calls "continuously acting antibiosenescent processes." These include free-radical scavengers, antioxidants, DNA repair and so forth. Genetic engineering of the regulatory genes is too complex at the present time, so Cutler found a short cut: trick the cells with something like an anti-aging vaccine. One could inject a bit of "fake aging" and the body would alter its level of protective enzymes to combat this fake aging antibody. It works on a similar principle as the smallpox vaccine.

One could pop a pill that would diffuse into the cells and fool them into thinking "Hey, we've got a lot of DNA damage." The cells, consequently, might raise the level of DNA repair enzyme to match the needs of a longer-lived organism. "We might be able to stimulate a whole battery of repair processes," Cutler speculates, "by inserting a highly damaged piece of DNA, with everything imaginable wrong with it. And all the repair mechanisms would be stimulated by the artifact. You don't even have to know how it works to use it."

LOOK OF THE FUTURE

Cutler, unlike many gerontologists, has been willing to speculate a bit on the nature of *Homo longevus*. He says: "My guess is that it would be best, not only to double man's maximum lifespan potential, but also to double his brain size. Although doubling size is not likely to improve the quality of the brain, it might provide a greater redundant capacity for neurons and their supporting cells, thereby, perhaps, delaying the onset of senility even further."

By reducing a person's growth rate by one-half and doubling the time for the brain's development and maturation (its growth rate would remain the same as now, and only one extra division of cells is needed to double its size), one might grow up to be an adult who looked much like a 12-year-old of today in terms of body and brain-size proportion.

When will it happen? Science writer and author of the soon to be published *Life-Extension Handbook*, Saul Kent, believes predictions are irrelevant. "It's inevitable, but the timing depends completely on the effort. I could give you a sliding scale in years before the breakthrough, depending on the effort put into it."

"If life-extension becomes a national priority like the space program," says Paul Segall, "if the Americans, the Russians, and the Japanese join hands, if there were a $200 billion assault on aging and death, this could produce dramatic results in five years. Just $200 billion, involving tens of hundreds of scientists, hundreds of thousands of technicians—in five years we'd have a program that would put such a dent in death we might wipe if off the face of the earth. And a program such as this would cost no more than these countries are now spending on the maintenance of old age homes."

At present, however, there is no clear cut directive for life-extension research. The House Select Committee on Aging is holding hearings on the advisability of funding life-extension research. But as one committee member admitted privately, "we really don't know what we're doing. We don't know who to listen to."

Although NIA Director, Dr. Robert Butler, has officially stated that life-extension research is a "priority of the NIA," this priority is not reflected in the Gerontology Research Center's $7-million share of the total 1978 NIA budget of

$37.3 million. And the entire NIA budget, moreover, pales beside the National Institute on Cancer's $872 million for 1978. The irony is profound, especially as evidence mounts that cancer is predominately an age-related disease. There may be no way to cure cancer without curing aging.

"A lot of resistance to life-extension comes in the form of questions about over-crowding the planet, population explosions, social security, jobs, etc.," explains F. M. Esfandiary, a normative philosopher who teaches courses at New York's New School For Social Research. "At its base the question is pathological. After eons of programming to accept death, we suddenly find we can conquer death. As we're getting closer to vanquishing it, people are getting up-tight—Elizabeth Kübler-Ross is a case in point. They are afraid to face the idea they can beat death. They are afraid to be disappointed. We still don't have the infrastructure for life, but in the demise of religion, guilt-orientation, and orthodoxy, we're moving toward a life-orientation."

So prolonged lifespan is inevitable. But is it advisable? "It is impossible to foresee what it will do to society," says Roy Walford. "I think it will be highly destabilizing, and I'm in favor of that."

Lots of senile tricentenarians? Not so, says Rolf Martin, biochemist from the City University of New York. Martin designed a "survival curve" projecting that the proportion of nonproductive oldsters actually will be reduced by two-thirds if lifespan is doubled. People would die of other things before they got senile.

The biggest argument for life-extension, in some minds, is that the actual "advancement of civilization"—that sacred cow of the Western world—is imperiled by the exponential rise in knowledge.

The solution so far has been specialization. But as we become more and more specialized, our ability to communicate to people outside our field diminishes. Our awareness narrows. Fewer people are gifted with the ability to put it all together. We may simply require more time to learn.

"We need to investigate why man's lifespan evolved in the first place," Cutler says. "Because that is what made man what he is today. A longer lifespan allowed man to make use of a larger brain, become more self-conscious, see the world and learn. It is difficult for me to see why a continuation along the same lines wouldn't result in more of the benefits that accrued in the first place.

"In reality, the slowing down and cessation of the evolution of a longer lifespan might have been an artifact, a negative by-product of increasing civilization, and was, in a sense, *abnormal*. Continued self-evolution of extended lifespan and intelligence is getting back to the biological norm—getting back on the road again."

Says Cutler: "If you ask me about the ethics of extending our lifespan along evolutionary lines, I must say that, if we do not evolve a longer lifespan—that is unethical."

A TEST OF AGE

by Dr. Bernard Dixon

Old many years before his time. . .Everlastingly youthful . . . Looks twenty years younger . . . Shows her years . . . Has the secret of eternal youth . . . Aged quite remarkably while in office.

Clichés or accurate comments? Do we really grow old at different rates? Does the biological clock tick more slowly for some people than for others? If so, what influence might one's occupation have on its timekeeping? These are some of the many intriguing questions posed by the science of aging. Until recently there was no satisfactory way of attempting to answer these questions. Now, as a result of research carried out at the University of Jyväskylä, in Finland, we have an interesting new technique that may provide answers.

Dr. Anja Kiiskinen and his colleagues became concerned with aging as a result of their work in occupational health. Some jobs, as everyone

33

knows, are less healthy and more tiring than others. But could it be that onerous occupations actually age employees prematurely?

There is no single factor, such as blood pressure, that may be measured to give an unambiguous answer. What we can do, however, is use a battery of different indices, all of them associated with aging, to calculate the "functional capacity" of a person being tested. If, for example, we assess an individual's grip strength *and* nearsightedness *and* breathing capacity *and* a range of other aptitudes, the combined results provide a measure of his or her functional capacity. This is certainly related to chronological age because, whatever our personal strengths and weaknesses, the aggregate score worsens as we get older. In other words, the so-called functional capacity provides us with a single numerical measurement that can be used in order to rate a person's bodily well-being.

The secret of Dr. Kiiskinen's research is the way in which he uses measurements of functional capacity. He simply compares it, person for person, with chronological age. The resulting ratio provides an entirely new measure known as "functional age." It is an indicator of our real, as opposed to our expected, bodily capacities. On this basis, Kiiskinen's results show that some of us are indeed younger, or older, than our calendar years suggest.

Workers at several Finnish refining factories were assessed by this method. Persons under thirty-three years of age and those over fifty-two were studied; they included blue-collar employees doing foundry work and white-collar employees in planning and administration. More than 300 people took part in the survey, and all underwent tests of their senses, blood circulation, muscles, lungs, and central nervous system. Kiiskinen's team then calculated mean values of the results for managerial, skilled, and semiskilled groups.

The outcome, as reported in *IRCS Medical Science* (1981, Vol. 9, p. 6), is fascinating. The average functional age of managerial types is indeed better—for both sexes—than that of skilled and semiskilled employees. More detailed analysis shows that a low (young) functional age in men is associated with longer education, higher income, and lighter and more interesting work. For women, the important factors are longer education and physically active leisure time. Particularly revealing is the influence of socioeconomic status and education. In all three groups this correlates more strongly with chronological age than with either health status or living habits.

Whenever a public figure dies in office, we hear that the pressure of his job was to blame. History does not support this view. Since 1850, for example, only one British prime minister has died before the age of seventy. Seven passed the age of eighty, and Churchill was over ninety.

Kiiskinen's studies illuminate this paradox. The last group to show signs of premature bodily wear and tear is that of well-educated, middleclass managers and administrators. We have to look elsewhere, in this case to nonmanagerial employees of Finland's metal-refining industry, for unambiguous evidence of accelerated aging. There may be lessons in this research for all of us.

SUPERPOWDER

by Albert Rosenfeld

The black mice in two cages, side by side, stir up memories of ancient fables. Those in one cage are sleek and healthy. Those in the other appear fatter and older. Yet all the mice are the same age and the same breed, like siblings in a venerable morality tale about the rewards of good living and the wages of dissoluteness.

In fact, the story of these mice is more dramatic than a fable. Both sets of mice at Temple University's Fels Research Institute, in Philadelphia, are in potentially grave danger. All have inherited susceptibility to a serious disease that causes their antibodies, meant to attack invading microorganisms, to kill their own blood cells instead. The fatter mice are developing anemia as a result of this genetic affliction. Chances are, they will die from it. The slim and healthy animals are protected by a white, powdery substance sprinkled liberally on their food. The substance, a hormone called DHEA, is prolonging their lives.

Medical researchers since Hippocrates have sought the magic bullet to cure all ills. No one is claiming that DHEA is it. But early returns from research suggest that this natural hormone, whose full name is dehydroepiandrosterone, may

37

be able to hit multiple targets with a single shot.

Biochemist Arthur G. Schwartz, master of the Temple mice, points out that DHEA seems to counter obesity as well as protect the lab animals from their genetic disease. The slender, scholarly scientist is not given to overstatement. But Schwartz says the hormone might very well work on humans, too. DHEA could also help combat diabetes, prevent cancer, and safeguard the cardiovascular system from heart attack or stroke, Schwartz says. It might even provide a firstline defense against aging.

Consider just one effect of DHEA. It inhibits the production or function of an enzyme called G-6-PD (glucose-6-phosphate dehydrogenase), which is essential to the body's use of sugar. Any substance that can interfere with this metabolic "pathway" is bound to affect a number of the body's important functions, including cell division. It is not at all amazing that a G-6-PD inhibitor would have varied uses. Besides, DHEA influences other biochemical pathways that relate to such vital processes as fatty-acid metabolism and the making of DNA, the molecular basis of heredity. So versatility is built right into it.

The relative obscurity of DHEA outside the scientific community may seem strange in view of its abundance in our bodies. For example, it is something like 20 times as plentiful in our blood as the hormone cortisone — which, like DHEA, is made by the adrenal glands, two inch-wide glands, one atop each kidney. And the population of DHEA molecules in the circulation on a given day may outnumber a thousandfold those of the sex hormones. Yet, though most of us are familiar with all those estrogens and androgens despite their sparsity, few of us have ever heard of DHEA.

The main problem has been to define DHEA's primary biological role. For a long time there was reluctance even to recognize it as a hormone. "You still won't find unanimity on that score among endocrinologists," Schwartz says.

DHEA does not act like most hormones and is, in fact, hard to find stored in the adrenals themselves. It seems to be released into the bloodstream as soon as it is manufactured. Another source of confusion is that DHEA can act as a precursor (forerunner) of the sex hormones. Yet that could scarcely be its main purpose. Why would so much of it be needed to make such tiny quantities of estrogens and androgens? DHEA can also be a metabolite, a leftover product of other hormonal reactions, and some have speculated that DHEA is merely a "waste steroid," a useless by-product bound for excretion.

Indeed DHEA is excreted in quantity. Nevertheless, researchers have found it in the testis, the ovary, the placenta, the fetus, and the lungs. And now the pioneering French investigator Etienne-Emile Baulieu, of the University of Paris, has extracted DHEA from the brains of rodents and primates — where, he believes, it is produced locally rather than imported from the adrenals. DHEA, he believes, can thus hardly be thought of as a mere waste product.

Rather, says biochemist Norman Applezweig, who runs his own New York consulting firm, "DHEA must have a role in the living system, one that has thus far eluded us." He suspects that DHEA will prove to be nothing less than a "regulator of metabolism in health and disease." As he points out, DHEA has already been tried as therapy — mostly in Europe — for a variety of human diseases, among them psoriasis, osteoporosis (a disease in which bones lose their calcium), gout, depression, hypertension, diabetes, and the disorders of menopause. But "the results were questioned and in almost every case were attributed to the conversion of DHEA, somewhere in the body, to male or female hormones." With new approaches to testing, and new understanding of DHEA's mechanisms, however, Applezweig is convinced that it may well become the most important drug of its kind ever to be developed.

Most of the studies in this country have been carried out, so far, in animals. But clinicians who know of DHEA's potential — especially in breast cancer, obesity, and diabetes — are itching to start human tests.

Spearheading the new investigative thrust is Arthur Schwartz's group at Temple. Like many research scientists, Schwartz was initially attracted by the mysteries surrounding DHEA. Why should the adrenals secrete the substance in such generous quantities? He was especially fascinated by studies carried out in the 1950's indicating that DHEA production reaches its peak at the age of about twenty-five, then declines steadily. Research by Claude Migeon at Johns Hopkins, by birth-control-pill pioneer Gregory Pincus, and by a team of investigators in Japan show that toward the end of life, DHEA levels have diminished to 5 percent of these peak values. Such a dramatic, steady decline is unheard of among such hormones. Why does DHEA decline?

There were other curious pieces to the puzzle. Schwartz was drawn to a series of articles that appeared in the 1970's, mostly in British medical journals, reporting the results of a still-ongoing investigation of breast cancer in women by scientists at London's Imperial Cancer Research Fund. What particularly caught Schwartz's eye in these studies headed by cancer specialist Richard D. Bulbrook was the fact that DHEA was consistently below normal in women with breast cancer as well as in women who were predestined to develop breast cancer.

One never knows, in studying cancer, what is cause and what is effect. People with cancer lack normal levels of immune protection, for instance, and this might simply be one of the side effects of the disease. But a growing number of researchers believe that an impaired immune system is one of the preconditions permitting cancer to develop. Could the same be true of DHEA? If its absence or scarcity invariably accompanies breast cancer, might its presence be protective, or even therapeutic?

In the early 1970's Schwartz happened to be working with rat-liver cells in tissue culture. In this environment the cells are easily rendered malignant by dosing them with cancer-causing chemicals. He was looking for ways to prevent this transformation by protecting the cells with various steroid substances, members of a class of organic compounds, including various hormones. Why did Schwartz focus on steroids? "Well," Schwartz explains, "carcinogenic chemicals often look like steroids, structurally speaking. And in biochemistry there is a well-known phenomenon called competitive inhibition. Molecule A may cause a certain reaction. Molecule B, if it is sufficiently similar, will compete successfully, even preferentially, to react before A does. Thus, A will be inhibited from carrying out its 'intentions.' For this reason, drug companies often look for a substance that is similar in structure. And that was my idea—to find a similar steroid that would competitively inhibit the carcinogen and leave the cells normal.

"So when I saw Bulbrook's paper connecting DHEA with breast-cancer inhibition, I quickly got hold of some DHEA—for the wrong reason, as I now know. DHEA works not by competitive inhibition but by blocking G-6-PD [the enzyme that regulates sugar metabolism]. Nevertheless, it did work. With DHEA in the culture, the cells were protected. They didn't turn cancerous."

Schwartz soon moved from tissue cultures to animal cancer studies of his own. Then in 1977 another provocative DHEA paper appeared. Terence T. Yen, a biochemist working in the pharmaceutical labs of Eli Lilly and Company, in Indianapolis, tried DHEA in mice especially bred to be obese, and he found that their weight dropped significantly.

Here was another riddle: Could it be that DHEA simply killed their appetite? In many classic studies where calories had been severely restricted (though nutritional balance was maintained) to extend the lifespan of laboratory rodents, the animals were also less obese and less cancer-prone. Could the effects of DHEA result simply from eating less? Yen quickly ascertained that the mice on DHEA did not suffer any loss of appetite. They ate as much as their litter mates, which, without DHEA, got much fatter.

Schwartz's own animal experiments soon confirmed both the antiobesity and anticancer effects of DHEA. The substance slimmed down fat rodents. And in mice genetically predisposed to develop spontaneous breast cancer, DHEA inhibited tumor formation, he discovered. Despite the large doses he administered over the course of a full year—more than ten times as much as the amount of cortisone he would have dared to give, for instance, even to a rodent—there were no apparent toxic effects. "It's much too early of course in the game to feel confident about safety," Schwartz warns.

What, for instance, might go wrong? For one thing, since DHEA *is* a precursor of the sex hormones, some scientists believe it might be damaging to the reproductive organs of both females and males, even perhaps incurring the risk of uterine or prostate cancer. If that came to pass, the well-meaning doctor would have caused cancer while trying to prevent it. Biochemist Norman Applezweig doubts that this would happen. "In very obese people," he says, "as well as in patients with cancer or diabetes, or for that matter in any of us who are growing older, DHEA has fallen below, often far below, its optimal level. So we would merely be giving replacement doses to get DHEA back up to where it ideally ought to be."

Applezweig of course recognizes that logic is no guarantee of safety. "Any substance could have unforeseen, and perhaps serious, side effects once it is put into widespread use. We've seen it happen with all too many drugs, and it could of course turn out to be true of DHEA as well. We'll never know until we give it a good try."

Applezweig and Schwartz are not the only people eager to give it that good try. One of Schwartz's collaborators is nutritional biochemist Margot Cleary, of Drexel University, also in Philadelphia. She's done obesity studies on mice and on normal-weight rats as well as rats genetically bred for obesity. In all cases the food intake has remained essentially the same. And in all cases less weight was put on with DHEA in the food than without it. Cleary found that in every case (though in varying quantities) the overall amount of fat tissue went down, but so did the size of individual fat cells. When she merely restricted the amount of food, there was no alteration in the body fat-cell size. This seems to clinch the argument for the antifat properties of DHEA and suggests why other researchers believe that DHEA will also be useful in preventing cardiovascular disease. Researchers have long recognized that fat metabolism can play a major role in warding off heart and vascular disorders and strokes.

Another researcher specializing in fat mice is biochemist Douglas Coleman, of the Jackson Laboratory, in Bar Harbor, Maine. His purebred strains of mice are not only obese but also diabetic. Though he has been experimenting with DHEA for only a short time, the usually conservative Coleman has already noted "remarkable effects, both dramatic and obvious." Coleman has worked with his genetically obese mice for many years, and he knows they tend to stay fat even when he cuts their food rations in half. Yet, on DHEA, eating their full diet, one grossly obese group of mice gained weight much less rapidly. More impressive, the diabetic mice, even those that fail to respond to insulin therapy, *do* respond to DHEA. Their blood sugar drops to normal. And these sick and susceptible mice that usually die at the age of six months "seem to go on indefinitely — at least another six months that we know of so far — once they are put on DHEA." So in these instances DHEA has doubled the life expectancy of these short-lived animals. Unfortunately, such experiments in rats and mice are not reliably translatable to human beings, especially in cancer research. And, as the French researcher Baulieu has taken pains to point out, DHEA metabolism is not the same in rodents as in humans.

Nevertheless, recalling Bulbrook's studies of Englishwomen with breast cancer, Schwartz believes that DHEA should be tried. And he says that a number of cancer clinicians—notably at Houston's M. D. Anderson Hospital and at New York's Memorial Sloan-Kettering Cancer Center—stand ready to go ahead once all the preliminary obstacles have been cleared.

What are those obstacles? One is a lack of money. Drug companies, even Eli Lilly, where Yen did his antiobesity experiments, have shown little interest in funding the work, in part because DHEA is not a patentable substance. But this objection could be overcome if DHEA lives up to even a fraction of its promise. And Schwartz says that synthetic analogs of the substance—with slightly altered molecules retaining DHEA's beneficial effects—would be patentable. The search for such commercially attractive analogs is on. In fact Schwartz is already working with one whose effects seem, in early trials, to be superior to DHEA's.

Schwartz believes financial support will be forthcoming shortly. And then the human tests known as "Phase I trials," undertaken just to prove safety, could be promptly carried out. But after that it will require many months of testing in animals (in rodents at first; then at least 90 days of further testing in nonrodents, dogs, for example). By the time all this clears through the Food and Drug Administration, perhaps a year will have passed. Then clinical trials in larger numbers of people, to prove efficacy as well as to confirm safety, will take another few years. So it's unlikely that DHEA will be available for general human use until nearly the end of the decade.

The first trials that Schwartz and his clinical collaborators would undertake would be an attempt to prevent or retard the growth of cancers. (Schwartz has seen no evidence so far that DHEA would be effective in treating cancers that were already established.) Who might the first subjects be?

"In the human female," Schwartz says, "obesity is known to be a predisposing factor in breast cancer. A high-fat diet also seems to elevate the risk. In view of the link between excess fat and breast cancer, and deducing from the experimental findings obtained so far, it is reasonable to guess that DHEA ought to be a useful preventive. One of the first clinical trials might enlist women who are vulnerable because of their family history."

Is breast cancer the only type of malignancy DHEA protects against? Schwartz thinks not. One breed of laboratory mouse, for instance, is susceptible to artificially induced cancer. If you put a carcinogen on the skin, then add another substance called a "promoter," skin cancer quickly develops. But if you give mice a single dose of DHEA, simply applying it to the skin before you apply the promoter, the carcinogen's action is blocked, and no tumor forms. "Since many substances in the environment are suspected of being cancer promoters," Schwartz suggests, "it's possible that DHEA might protect against them."

Certain kinds of chemically induced lung and colon cancer in mice have also been shown by

Schwartz's team to be inhibited by DHEA. So those at high risk of developing colon cancer would also be on Schwartz's list of people who would be included in the first clinical trials of DHEA. One final experiment: A common African cancer called Burkitt's lymphoma — a cancer of the lymphatic tissue — is caused by the Epstein-Barr virus, transmitted by insects. In tissue culture, this virus can also transform human white blood cells into cancerous cells. But when DHEA is added to the mix, this transformation does not take place. In sum, DHEA has already demonstrated possible effectiveness in preventing cancers of the breast, liver, skin, colon, and lungs, as well as Burkitt's lymphoma. And the testing has barely begun.

Researchers in many places have recorded suggestive evidence for DHEA's other multifarious effects. Carolyn Berdanier, of the University of Georgia, working with rats that age and sicken prematurely, found that DHEA gave them more energy and held down fat production. Vernon Riley, of the Pacific Northwest Research Foundation, in Seattle, demonstrated DHEA's striking antistress effects. M. Ben-David, at Hebrew University, in Jerusalem, used DHEA to bring down cholesterol levels, again in rodents. Baulieu has even proposed that there should be clinical trials of DHEA for schizophrenics.

Most interesting, perhaps, is a series of experiments carried out by a team of Hungarian scientists in Prague, led by Jiri Sonka, of Karlova University. Noting, as others had, that the decline of DHEA coincides with a host of degenerative disorders, Sonka theorized that as DHEA's inhibiting effects wane with age, destructive processes are allowed to flourish unchecked. The result is what he calls "the hyperproductive syndrome." Taking a hard look at a number of elderly patients suffering from obesity, hypertension, heart troubles, cirrhosis, and gout, and finding their levels of DHEA low both in blood and in urine, Sonka put them on varying dosages of DHEA.

He was able to raise DHEA levels, and claimed noticeable improvement in all except the gout victims, whose elevated uric-acid levels went even higher instead of coming down as expected. But Sonka worked with only a small number of patients and used no "matched controls." Besides, too many other things were happening to those patients at the same time for him to be sure the good effects were due solely to DHEA. So his results have not been taken very seriously. But they were interesting enough to suggest the need for more clinical work.

All this has led Applezweig to the conclusion that, unlike most hormones, which *excite* (the word *hormone* comes from a Greek word meaning "to stir up") cells into activity, DHEA rather acts to "deexcite" metabolic processes. So DHEA behaves more like an antihormone. "If insufficiency of DHEA leads to runaway production of nucleic acids, fats, and hormones, then replacement therapy with DHEA should curb those excesses that manifest themselves in the diseases of aging."

Schwartz, who can't help noticing that all his animals on DHEA seem to look younger than those that are not, agrees that DHEA may well be effective in staving off some of the more serious ravages of aging. In fact, it was this possibility that brought Schwartz and DHEA to the attention of the private, nonprofit Fund for Integrative Biomedical Research, with a special interest in aging—or, rather, antiaging. The scientific director of the Washington, D.C.-based foundation, cancer specialist William Regelson, of the Medical College of Virginia, has taken a personal hand in accelerating DHEA research.

"Even if DHEA turns out to have no direct impact on the aging process itself," Regelson says, "it does seem to hold back so many of the individual degenerative processes that, barring some terrible unforeseen effects, I think DHEA is bound to improve the quality of our later years."

In the short term these benefits will depend on obtaining large quantities of standardized DHEA to carry out the remaining research. While awaiting the arrival of the synthetic form, investigators have turned to a lowly Mexican yam. Natives call it *barbasco*. Its Latin name is *Dioscorea floribunda,* a deceptively romantic name for a poisonous plant—with some useful medical properties. You'll never find it in the supermarket, but the yam provided the original raw materials for the first birth-control steroids. And it can be processed to produce DHEA, a fact well-known to Mexican government officials. Faced with the prospect of opening up a huge market for the *barbasco,* they would like to see research and clinical trials carried out with dispatch. In fact Mexico may sponsor some trials with or without American collaboration.

DHEA is already better known south of the border than in the United States. Applezweig, who has served as a consultant for the Mexican government, recalls that only a few months ago the head of the Mexican research agency, Proquivimex, inadvertently caused a sensation. He granted the request of a prominent TV commentator, whose dog was stricken with breast cancer, for a supply of DHEA. On large doses of the hormone, the dog apparently made a strong comeback after surgery. Mexico's national television network played up the story, and it caused a stir among viewers.

The real news is more spectacular. Without surgery or side effect, dozens of mice and rats have now defeated several diseases, their defenses bolstered by a multiple-target drug. And researchers suggest that these stories of rodent success may foreshadow new human victories over an array of ancient enemies.

PART TWO:
DIET DISCOVERIES

NUTRITION HYPE

By Daniel Greenberg

Sometime within the next few years, a food manufacturing company will announce the development of a new snack food. It might be a chocolate-covered cupcake or a milk shake or a candy bar—it could come in almost any form. But the feature the food company will advertise most prominently is that this snack, though composed mostly of refined sugar, will be *nutritious*. That is, by eating just one cupcake, milk shake, or whatever, you will be meeting the U. S. Recommended Daily Allowances (RDAs) for every nutrient considered vital to good health by the Food and Drug Administration (FDA).

It's not such a farfetched idea. We're currently in the middle of a "fortification war" in which the widely touted U. S. RDAs for protein and 19 vitamins and minerals have become major weapons in the hands of the food company giants. Any foods that can proudly display on the sides of their glossy packages that they meet 100 percent of any or all of the RDAs instantly gain a tremendous advantage over their competition on the supermarket shelves.

The future implications of the fortification wars are far from optimistic, however. True, the promise of getting all of one's Recommended

Daily Allowances from a single snack is indeed inviting. But the cruel reality is that it's possible to consume 100 percent of every one of the 20 RDAs and still starve to death. Or at least be seriously malnourished.

The RDA standard may be one of the single largest obstacles to the future of healthful nutrition in this country. It is outdated, vulnerable to exploitation, and basically useless in guiding Americans toward a healthy diet. What's worse, it can be misleading. Consumers are convinced that the RDAs reflect scientific knowledge of sound nutrition and dine under the illusion that eating a full share of RDAs is the key to health.

It's simply not true. Despite advertising claims to the contrary, adding up RDA percentages on the labels of processed foods until you reach 100 percent for every nutrient (protein, iron, calcium, copper, iodine, magnesium, phosphorus, zinc, biotin, niacin, thiamin, riboflavin, folic acid, pantothenic acid, and vitamins A, C, D, E, B_6, and B_{12}) is just not the way to eat.

Here, then, are the unfortified and unappetizing facts on our U. S. RDA system and why it doesn't work.

AN IDEA WHOSE TIME HAS GONE

The RDAs may have been useful back in the 1940s for combating deficiency diseases such as rickets, pellagra, and scurvy, but these problems are almost nonexistent in present-day America. Instead, we are faced with the problem of excess, particularly in regard to sugar, fats, and salt, all of which can be detrimental to health when ingested in large quantities. The RDA system not only remains oblivious of the harm these substances may cause but, ironically, tends to encourage their consumption. For example, many popular cereals are heavily fortified so as to provide 100 percent or more of many RDAs. But they are also heavily laced or coated with sugar to make them more palatable. The consumer gets the impression that he's eating well, when in fact his excess intake of sugar is subjecting him to many health hazards.

And recently, in a government-supported food program for women, children, and infants, a cereal containing 68 percent sugar was allowed while more healthful cereals — those that were whole-grain and lower in sugar content, such as oatmeal and shredded wheat — were not allowed, simply because they contained less than 45 percent of the RDA for iron.

Where do the RDAs come from? Like so much else in the scientific realm, the RDA system can be traced back to military considerations. At the beginning of World War II, concern over the adequacy of the national food supply turned government attention to the question of what the nutritional requirements of the American people are. In 1943, the nation's most prestigious scientific society, the National Academy of Sciences (NAS), agreed to take on the job. Today, as they did then, the RDA ratings originate in the academy's Food and Nutrition Board, composed of learned figures in the nutritional sciences. Every five years the board reviews the latest scientific literature and produces a publication, *Recommended Dietary Allowances*. This, plus other sources, is in turn used by the FDA to calculate the U. S. Recommended *Daily* Allowances that show up on your food packages.

But despite the elaborate procedures set up to

create the RDAs, there are still many holes in the system. For example, it ignores many nutrients, at least 20, that have been identified as essential to good health.

This policy can have far-reaching effects on the public health. Bonnie F. Liebman, a consumer representative on the Food and Nutrition Board, recently told a congressional inquiry about some of the abuses. Ms. Liebman explained that hospital dieticians, as well as many other institutional food planners, are often so obsessed with the RDA system that they tend to disregard other nutritional factors, just so long as they can pack those RDAs into their meal planning. "Because of the availability of highly processed, highly fortified food products," she said, "they [the dieticians] can easily overlook the presence or absence of other dietary constituents, such as fat, saturated fat, trace elements, and fiber, which now pose far greater public-health problems than those nutrients included in the RDA."

The problem is twofold: The RDA system ignores the modern need for more fiber, trace elements, and other nutrients in the diet while it indirectly encourages unhealthy intakes of sugars and fats.

So what kind of diet *should* the NAS and FDA be encouraging? That, we'll soon see, is yet another problem.

WHO KNOWS?

Nobody knows what a good diet is. Two years ago, the General Accounting Office (GAO), which conducts investigations for the U. S. Congress, made an extensive survey of the nutritional sciences. They went so far as to interview 32 leading nutrition researchers. The results? The GAO dourly concluded: "Given the present state of nutrition knowledge, it is not possible to say what constitutes an adequate diet."

And then there's the expert and gloomy appraisal of the nutrition sciences offered by Ross H. Hall, professor of biochemistry at McMaster University, Ontario, Canada: "The science of nutrition has essentially stagnated since the early 1950s, when the last vitamin to be discovered was announced." Yet during this time, Hall points out, monumental changes have occurred in the American food supply, to the point where factory-processed foods dominate the nation's diet. Whether this is good or bad, Hall insists, is unknown, because the nutritional sciences are hooked on the obsolete notion that by identifying RDA requirements, they are pointing the way to good nutrition.

THOSE MAGIC NUMBERS

Despite the credentials of the NAS and the FDA, there's nothing scientific about the RDA's magic numbers. On what basis, for example, does the FDA list six micromilligrams as the RDA for Vitamin B_{12} or 400 international units (IUs) as the RDA for Vitamin D? Also curious is that only one number is ever given for a particular nutrient on food-package labels, regardless of whether the consumer is a growing adolescent, a sedentary senior citizen, or a hardworking manual laborer. Surely requirements must differ among individuals according to age, activity, and sex. As a matter of fact, the academy's tables recognize these differences by establishing five age groups of males, females, and pregnant and lactating women. And each group is further divided by weight, height, and daily energy expenditure. But

the version the public gets—the FDA's RDAs—
gives only one amount for each nutrient. And
this is for "adults," defined by the FDA as anyone
over age four! (To be fair, the FDA does prescribe
different amounts for infants, children under age
four, and pregnant and lactating women, in its
public—but rarely seen—literature.)

Finally, if the RDAs are based on scientific
study, why is it that other nations have come out
with different numbers? In the U. S., for example, the adult RDA for Vitamin C is 45 milligrams
whereas in Canada and Britain it's 30; in West
Germany it's 75.

ENOUGH IS TOO MUCH

The RDAs are much too high. Since they originated because of wartime concern over nutritional adequacy, and at a time when the nutrition
sciences were most concerned with deficiency diseases, the whole thrust was toward making sure
the American population as a whole would get
essential nutrients. Since the focus was on the
masses, the single figure for each RDA had to be
set high above the average requirement to make
sure *everyone* got enough.

What the NAS and FDA strive for, then, are
RDAs set above the average requirements by
twice the standard deviation. Which means that
approximately 97.5 percent of our population
needs less than the specified RDA for any particular nutrient.

Stated otherwise, the system deems it better for
most of us to have too much than for some of us
to have too little. Once again, this reflects the an-
tiquated obsession with deficiency diseases, even
though for the most part they've long since disappeared from the land.

FAULTY TESTS

RDA tests are suspect. Strangely enough, the academy committee that periodically reissues the RDA tables admits that the scientific underpinnings for its recommendations are often pretty wobbly.

"Unfortunately," states the committee, "experiments on man are costly; they must often be of long duration; certain types of experiments are not possible for ethical reasons, and even under the best conditions only a small number of subjects can be studied in a single experiment. Thus, requirement estimates must often be derived from limited information."

Even when the RDAs are based on extensive experimentation, one of the most common techniques used — called "balance studies" — has been the subject of skepticism. Based on the assumption that when the body has enough of a nutrient, the surplus will be excreted, these studies are simply feed-and-measure exercises. What researchers look for is the amount that must be ingested to produce a surplus, from which, presumably, the minimum required for good nutrition can be calculated.

But these retention rates may have no significance so far as nutritional requirements are concerned, according to D. M. Hegsted, who recently left the Harvard School of Public Health to head the Department of Agriculture's newly established Human Nutrition Center. The rates, he observed in an article in the *Journal of Nutrition,* appear to vary without explanation when such factors as temperature and dosage are changed. Hegsted concluded that new analytical techniques are needed, and "until such methods are available, the results obtained with balance methods must be viewed with skepticism."

PROMOTING HUCKSTERISM

Besides creating an atmosphere of scientific certainty, when in fact much of the scientific basis behind it is pretty shaky, the RDA system also lends itself to hucksterism.

In their early days, the RDA ratings were mainly of interest only to government planners and various technocrats. But as the vitamin craze developed in postwar America, food manufacturers began to realize that RDAs could be a potent marketing tool. And in 1974, when the FDA instituted a requirement for nutritional labeling on most packaged foods, the fortification wars began in earnest, with manufacturers competing to outdo each other in providing — and even exceeding — the government-certified Recommended Daily Allowances. Toward this goal, they were prodded on by manufacturers of vitamin and mineral supplements, who heavily advertised in the trade press about the marketing wallop to be had with high RDAs.

It is interesting to note that a possible by-product of the fortification war is that Americans are eating less fresh fruit and vegetables than ever before. While fruits and vegetables are valuable sources of a majority of the nutrients on the RDA list, RDAs are listed on packaged foods only. Which gives Kellogg's cornflakes a distinct advertising edge over corn on the cob.

LABEL OF THE FUTURE

The problem of what to do about the system has been rumbling around government circles and the food industry for years. RDA ratings *can* be defended on the ground that poor as they are they represent the best available knowledge and are therefore valuable guides, if properly used. In response to the argument that label information is too sparse to be meaningful to the average consumer, the industry counters that it would take a label the size of a newspaper page to provide full details about nutrient content and requirements.

Yet some have proposed that the present labeling be replaced with simple charts that would concentrate on such basics as roughage, salt, sugar, fats, proteins, and carbohydrates — leaving out the currently listed RDA items on the assumption that any reasonably diversified diet will probably provide all of them.

It is very likely that we will see major changes in food-product labeling within five years, if not sooner — because one of the advocates of more comprehensible labeling is Donald Kennedy himself, commissioner of the FDA. One possibility might be a pie-shaped graph, which would quickly show how much of a product was made up of sugar, protein, salt, and so on. Another chart might spell out daily nutritional needs based on weight and height, as opposed to the current system of a single standard for everyone.

And perhaps the FDA may break its fixation with minimum requirements for "good" nutrients and concentrate more on *maximum* allowances for potentially harmful substances like sugar and fat. In which case we may see a new "anti-fortification war" in which food companies scramble to get their products in *under* these new requirements.

Meanwhile, for a public that's increasingly befuddled by a wildly conflicting nutritional clamor, the best advice is to eat sparingly from a wide variety of foods — particularly fresh ones — and don't pay too much attention to RDAs. In any sensible diet it's hard to avoid them.

NUTRITION FADS AND FALLACIES

The mere fact that no one knows what good nutrition really is hasn't kept enthusiasts, faddists, and outright quacks from spreading ill-founded diets among the American public.

One of the country's most influential faddists was the Reverend Sylvester W. Graham, who claimed that meats and fats inflame sexual desires — and were therefore to be avoided. Mustard, catsup, and pepper, he said, cause insanity.

One of his prominent followers was Dr. John Harvey Kellogg, manager of the Battle Creek (Michigan) Sanitarium, which treated almost any illness with diets Graham had prescribed.

Dr. Kellogg invented a cereal called Granose, which sold 100,000 pounds its first year. His company now accounts for over 40 percent of the breakfast-food business in the U. S. One of its major competitors was founded by C. W. Post after a nine-month stay at the sanitarium.

A less successful "nutritionist" was Adolphus Hohensee, who set himself up as a physician and nutrition expert in the 1940s. His professional qualifications were one semester of high school and a carnival barker's sense of salesmanship.

The average American diet, Hohensee declared, could ruin the kidneys, blood, veins, and intestines. His diet, he claimed, could restore all bodily organs except the kidneys, dissolving "incrustations" in the brain and eyes that block clear thinking and clear vision, and helping its followers live to be 180.

In 1948, Hohensee was arrested in Phoenix

and fined $1800 for his fraud. He was convicted again six years later, in Scranton, Pennsylvania. While his case was pending appeal, news photographers caught him in a Houston restaurant, pouring down beer and eating both fried red snapper and white bread.

Then there was Gaylord Hauser, who claimed that most people over 40 suffer malnutrition, a cause of "premature aging." The cure for this, he said, lay in such wonder foods as brewer's yeast, powdered skim milk, and blackstrap molasses.

Hauser's brand of dietary mythology sold well. His book *Look Younger, Live Longer* was third on the nonfiction bestseller list in 1950, first in 1951.

It's tempting to try to draw some profound conclusion from all this. Frankly, we haven't thought of any. As P. T. Barnum observed when the population was much smaller, there's a sucker born every minute. Claiming sure knowledge in the uncertain world of nutrition is one of the most reliable ways to part him from his money.

MIND FOOD

By Sandy Shaw and Durk Pearson

Picture it: It's time to learn a programming language for your new home computer. Your first step? A trip to the drugstore, of course. Learning to program a computer is too tough a job to take on without a good supply of your favorite "smart pills."

At the pharmacy, the shelf marked INTELLIGENCE BOOSTERS AND CREATIVITY EXPANDERS holds at least a dozen drugs. The pharmacist fills your order: 1,000 Hydergine tablets, 6 bottles of Diapid nasal spray, a kilogram of ribonucleic acid (RNA) powder, 100 grams of dl-phenylalanine, a gram of vitamin B_{12}, and a kilogram of Deaner tablets. You just carry the drugs home, take them on schedule, and promptly learn your new language with a lot more fun and a lot less pain than you'd have had before you found intelligence drugs.

There is nothing futuristic about this scenario.

The order is ours, and we're using it right now. The cooperative druggist may be a fantasy (Did he ask for a prescription?), but increasing brainpower is not.

This is a "how-to" article. You can actually use the drugs we are talking about to increase your own intelligence and creativity. We'll tell you how some of these drugs work, how to use them, and what effects and side effects to expect. Several of the compounds discussed here are vitamins or amino acids — nutrients that are generally exempt from government control and can be purchased freely. Others are prescription drugs approved by the Food and Drug Administration (FDA) for other purposes. A few cannot be had in this country for reasons we will go into later.

Keep in mind that none of these drugs has the FDA's approval for increasing normal intelligence, nor can they get it. The FDA approves only drugs that prevent or cure diseases. Intelligence boosters simply do not fit in their scheme of things. If you want to improve your mental powers, you will have to evaluate the drugs yourself.

Medical researchers have found more than a dozen chemicals* that promote intelligence — learning ability or data processing in standard-

---

*The list includes ribonucleic acid (RNA). Isoprinosine, vasopressin, Hydergine, Deaner, lecithin, choline, phenylalanine, amphetamines and related compounds, magnesium pemoline, diphenylhydantoin, Ritalin vitamin B_{12}, Nootropyl, $ACTH_{4-10}$, l-prolyll-leucyl glycine amide, caffeine, Metrazol, and strychnine. There are others, but these are the most interesting.

ized tasks—in animals and man. Many have also been used to reverse senile memory loss, depression, and other effects of aging. As the brain ages, it slowly loses its supply of neurotransmitters—chemicals that carry nerve impulses across the gap, or synapse, between one cell and another—or it becomes less sensitive to them. Doses of artificially supplied neurotransmitters, their biochemical precursors, and drugs that mimic them have all been used to replace the missing compounds, resulting in improved mental function. Even in young people, the supply of neurochemicals is limited, so the mental performance of young adults can also be substantially improved.

Each brain chemical has an optimum level, however. Above or below that amount, there's less improvement in intelligence, sometimes even a decline. The only way to find out what is best for you is by systematic experiments. Drug effects can be subtle at first, and you almost always need a learning period to recognize and use any improvement in memory or data processing.

The chemical details of learning and memory are not yet well understood, though knowledge in this area is expanding rapidly. According to current theories, several chemical systems are involved.

One of the most important neurotransmitters involved in memory and learning is acetylcholine, a compound that also plays major roles in motor and sensory control, long-term planning, and primitive drives and emotions. It is also one of the chemicals that show the sharpest declines in the aging brain. Drugs such as scopolamine, which inhibits acetylcholine activity in the brain, produce in young people a complex pattern of learning deficiencies resembling that of old age. Thus, the decline of acetylcholine activity is thought to be important in senile memory loss and other age-related learning defects.

There are several safe and effective ways to increase the brain's acetylcholine supply. Choline, the raw material from which acetylcholine is made, raises brain levels of the neurotransmitter in laboratory animals. In normal young people, an oral dose of ten grams of choline improves memory and serial learning. Choline is a nutrient found in meat, eggs, and fish, so it is exempt from FDA regulation and can be found in most health-food stores. A daily dose of three grams is reasonable for adults.

Choline does have one unfortunate side effect, however: Some people have gut bacteria that digest choline, which gives the user an unpleasant, fishy body odor. Eating a high-fiber diet or large amounts of yogurt often changes the intestinal flora enough to eliminate the problem.

Lecithin (phosphatidyl choline) raises the level of acetylcholine in the brain even more effectively than choline itself, and it can be expected to improve memory and learning in the same way. In one successful experiment, test subjects took 80 grams per day, just over three ounces, and improved their memories markedly. The lecithin sold in health-food stores usually contains large amounts of fat as well, so this can be a high-calorie way to raise your intelligence. Unlike choline, lecithin causes no body odor.

The prescription drug Deaner, known chemically as dimethylaminoethanol *p*-acetamidobenzoate, also raises acetylcholine levels and improves memory and learning in the aged and in hyperkinetic children. In fact, even the FDA approves it as "possibly effective" in the treatment of learning problems and hyperkinesis. In many cases Deaner has also helped or cured senile memory loss, apathy and depression.

In addition to raising acetylcholine levels, Deaner "washes away" a cellullar aging pigment called lipofuscin, a waste product that may interfere with the functioning of nerve cells. Dr. Richard Hochshild, a gerontologist with the Microwave Instrument Company, used Deaner to lengthen the mean life span of mice by 50 percent and their maximum life span by a third.

Another chemical basic to learning and memory is ribonucleic acid. In the early 1960s, Dr. James V. McConnell, a University of Michigan psychologist, tried an experiment in which he taught planarian worms to crawl through a maze, then ground them up and fed them to other flatworms. The cannibals, he found, learned to negotiate the same maze significantly faster than worms on a normal diet. When he trained them to run a different maze, however, it took them longer to master the lesson. It seemed to be the worms' RNA that caused the effect.

RNA itself is an effective memory booster in experimental animals, and such other intelligence drugs as orotic and inosinic acids work because the body converts them to RNA. Doses of two to ten grams a day are about right. (When you extrapolate from animal experiments to human use, drug doses should be chosen so that they represent equal percentages of the subject's daily dry-food intake. Do not assume that because a mouse weighs three ounces and you weigh 3,000 ounces you can take 1,000 times the mouse's drug dose. Small animals metabolize drugs far faster than large ones, so that the human dose for some drugs is actually smaller than that for mice. Calculating dosages as a percentage of dry-food intake usually compensates for this difference.)

In addition to its memory-enhancing effect, RNA protects against oxidizing chemicals that seem to be a major cause of aging and probably contribute to senility. In this, RNA supplements mimic many natural "maintenance" systems. Plants, for example, protect themselves against damage caused by oxidants formed by exposure to ultraviolet light with such antioxidants as beta carotene, the yellow pigment in carrots and other plants, and vitamins C and E. RNA supplements significantly slow the deterioration seen in old age. In one experiment, a daily dose of 25 milligrams extended the average life span of laboratory mice by 16 percent.

RNA does have some drawbacks, however. Because of its acidity, it can cause stomach upset. A little baking soda taken at the same time will prevent this. More seriously, nucleic-acid metabolism produces large amounts of uric acid as a waste product, and uric acid is the cause of gout. RNA can seriously worsen gout in people who already suffer from it and may even cause gout in those who already have high urate levels. The uric acid can precipitate as crystals in the joints and kidneys causing permanent damage and severe pain. Though 90 percent of gout patients are male, woman can also suffer from it. Have a uric-acid test before taking RNA and a month or so after you begin.

For all that, oral RNA is virtually harmless in people with normal uric-acid levels. Dr. Max Odens, a London physician, has given people up to 80 grams per day, and they've suffered no ill effects.

Many health-food stores carry RNA, but check the label before you buy. Yeast is about 6 percent RNA, but the plant's cell walls are so hard to digest that the body takes in very little. If a product contains less than 12 percent RNA, you are probably just buying overpriced yeast with little available nucleic acid.

The drug Isoprinosine contains inosine, a raw material the body can use to make RNA, coupled with dimethylaminoethanol, a molecule that helps the inosine pass through the blood-brain barrier, a membrane that prevents most chemicals from entering the brain. The drug increases nucleic-acid synthesis in the brain-cell polyribosomes, cellular factories where RNA copied from the DNA of the genes is translated into proteins. This is a key step in memory formation. Though marketed only as an antiviral agent that combats some strains of polio, flu, and herpes, Isoprinosine is a potent RNA booster. Dr. Paul Gordon, who developed the drug in the early 1960s, says it enhances learning efficiency, aids memory, improves behavioral organization, and increases organization and integration of perceptual information. Isoprinosine is available in Europe and Mexico, but, unfortunately, FDA regulations have barred its use here.

Vitamin B_{12} also stimulates RNA synthesis in the brain nerves. Its administration to rats increased their rate of learning. A dose of 1,000 micrograms per day is reasonable.

Yet another chemical vital to learning and memory is the neurotransmitter norepinephrine (NE). Learning ability is severely depressed by drugs that inhibit its synthesis or remove it from the brain. NE itself, on the other hand, improves memory.

When not carrying nerve signals from cell to cell, NE is stored in microscopic pouches known as synaptic transmitter vesicles. To transmit a nerve impulse, NE is secreted into the synapse, then returned to the vesicle. Such drugs as the amphetamines, Ritalin, and magnesium pemoline block NE from reentering the vesicle, thereby increasing the amount of neurotransmitter in the synapse. They also promote memory and improve learning in focusing and attention tasks, but this may occur because they are central nerve stimulants which raise activity levels rather than because of their effect on data-processing.

One disadvantage of these drugs is that they no longer improve learning ability once the nerves have released most of their NE; the body develops a tolerance to the drug until more NE is synthesized. Depression often occurs during this interval.

Phenylalanine, an amino acid found in meat and cheese, is a natural forerunner of NE and a very effective mood elevator and stimulant that does not deplete the body's supply of NE. Doses of 100 to 500 milligrams a day for two weeks completely eliminate the depression seen after amphetamine use. Phenylalanine sometimes raises blood pressure, however, so people with hypertension should start with small doses and increase them gradually, making sure that their blood pressure remains under control. Though not controlled by the FDA, this drug is not yet available in pharmacies or health-food stores. It must be purchased as an industrial chemical.

Vasopressin, also known as antidiuretic hormone, is produced by the pituitary gland. Its main task in the body is to regulate blood pressure and urine volume, but in the brain it is also a powerful stimulant of memory and learning. Cocaine and several other popular drugs release vasopressin from the pituitary, which may explain why cocaine improves learning in tasks that require focusing and concentration and enhances the memory and the ability to re-experience remembered emotions. On the other hand, nicotine, alcohol, and marijuana inhibit vasopressin release.

Medical researchers have found that 16 units per day of Diapid nasal spray, a synthetic version of vasopressin, restores memory to amnesia patients and improves attention, concentration, motor rapidity, and memory in men in their fifties and sixties. We have used up to 40 units per day and gained amazing improvements in memory and learning. We have also experienced prolonged and intensified orgasms, an effect not mentioned in the scientific literature!

Diapid has few side effects. Studies have found no effect on blood pressure and urine volume, even at doses of 16 units per day. Intestinal cramps and nasal irritation are occasionally seen. Angina patients sometimes develop heart pain when using Diapid, but this does not seem medically dangerous. Diapid remains effective as long as it is used and, unlike cocaine, does not cause depression when discontinued.

Hydergine, a very safe drug, is approved by the FDA for treatment of depression, confusion, unsociability, and dizziness in the elderly. Scientific reports show that it has many other uses. Hydergine is a chemical relative of LSD. Though it has no hallucinogenic effects, it produces a feeling of extreme clear-headedness typical of very low doses of LSD. Hydergine improves learning and memory, and it can relieve confusion, apathy, and forgetfulness in the aged. This takes up to several months, depending on the condition's severity.

The neurotransmitters deliver chemical messages between nerve cells. But within the cell a "second messenger" (cyclic AMP) delivers messages from the cell membrane to the nucleus. Hydergine controls the level of the second messenger inside brain cells. Caffeine is a stimulant with a closely related effect on the second messenger, but because the action of Hydergine is more selective, it doesn't cause a come-down or jitters like caffeine and increases intellectual performance over a much wider range of dosages and rates of administration. A mutant fruit fly, called the "dumb" fruit fly, has recently been discovered. It is dumb because there is a defect in its control of the level of the second messenger. Hydergine also increases protein synthesis in the brain.

The recommended dosage of Hydergine is three milligrams per day in this country, only a third of the dose used in Europe. The drug is nontoxic at these dosages, though nausea and headaches do occasionally occur.

Hydergine has several complex effects that may be even more important than its benefits to memory and mood. During anesthesia, drowning, and perhaps stroke, it protects the brain against damage due to lack of oxygen and blood glucose. For this reason, it is used routinely in Europe to prepare patients for surgery.

It also stimulates the growth of neurites, fine tendrils that grow from each nerve cell, or neuron, in large numbers and form a complex network of cross connections. Each neuron may be in contact with 100,000 other nerve cells through its neurites. These fibers are essential for learning and data processing, but their numbers fall off drastically with age. Until recently, scientists believed this loss was permanent. It turns out, however, that a hormone called nerve-growth factor stimulates regeneration of the neurites. Six months to two years of Hydergine therapy may also reverse this loss, acting by the same mechanism as the natural hormone. Unfortunately, many physicians try the drug on their patients for a few days or weeks and, seeing no immediate effect, give up.

Nootropyl, known chemically as 2-oxo-pyrrolidine acetamide, is a new intelligence booster made in Europe. A chemical analogue of the neurotransmitter gamma-aminobutyric acid, it seems to promote the flow of information between the right and left hemispheres of the brain, at least in rats and mice. In man, communication between the sides of the brain seems to cause flashes of creativity. Though Nootropyl's toxicity is very low, it is unlikely that the FDA will ever allow this remarkable drug into the United States. Improved hemispheric communication just isn't the sort of cause they are prepared to deal with!

Many of the experiments with intelligence promoters in animals have been performed with strychnine, which produces clear improvements in maze learning and in visual and spatial discrimination in rats. Strychnine is extremely toxic, however. Doses large enough to produce significant benefits carry with them a high danger of convulsions and even death. Two human-dosage forms of strychnine were sold about ten years ago. These drugs are no longer offered. Strychnine currently has no medical value; the recommended doses are too small for measurable effect, and large doses are very dangerous.

Most intelligence research has been done on memorization or computation, not on creative processes. One reason may be that there is little demand for creative people in government and industry, where drones are less likely to rock the boat.

IQ tests are concerned with memorization and computation rather than with creativity. It is possible to have a very high IQ and never think a novel thought. Some psychologists have reported that creative thinking is associated with so-called theta rhythms, a type of electrical activity in the brain. In rats, very low doses of strychnine and Metrazol promote theta activity. It has recently been reported that vasopressin also has this effect. In man, biofeedback can be used to increase theta rhythms, often resulting in novel, often dreamlike, thought patterns. Vasopressin and LSD increase theta in humans.

People have said that they are more creative under the influence of such drugs as marijuana, LSD, vasopressin, and the substituted phenethylamines, a group of chemicals related to amphetamine. So far, there is little evidence to support these claims, though it has been confirmed that LSD and vasopressin increase visualization and imagination, which are both parts of creativity. In one very interesting study, Dr. Alexander Shulgin, a chemist renowned among pharmaceutical experimenters for his ability to design intriguing new drugs, found that DOET, a substituted phenethylamine, dramatically increased creativity in people who already displayed it but that it did not for uncreative people. These drugs are not available, and the FDA cannot approve them under today's rules.

If you want to try the prescription drugs we've described, there are several ways to improve your chances. A doctor who is newly in practice is more likely to give you a prescription than an old-line physician is and may know more about experimental drugs. Buy a copy of the *Physician's Desk Reference*, a handbook that will tell you when to avoid a given drug and what side effects to expect. Ask your doctor to test your kidneys, liver, and basic metabolic functions before trying any new drug, and repeat these tests at least once a year. It will reassure your doctor that you are responsible enough to use the drugs and could prevent serious side effects.

Do not expect any doctor to be an expert on intelligence boosters. Physicians are not research scientists and seldom have the time to follow experimental reports. They find out about new drugs from the manufacturers, and drug companies are forbidden to give physicians research papers about uses the FDA has not approved even when the doctor asks for them. We know one physician who wanted to learn about Hydergine research. It took him three months of writing letters and making phone calls just to get the forms he needed to ask the FDA's permission to receive "unauthorized" research reports from the manufacturer. Fortunately, we are research scientists rather than physicians and had no trouble obtaining the literature. It seems strange that the FDA prevents the people who prescribe drugs from getting the information they need to make decisions.

We hope that this roadblock in the path to more powerful intellects will soon be eliminated. Data slowly filtering out of pharmaceutical laboratories have made it clear that current FDA regulations are blocking the development of valuable new drugs in many fields of reserach. A growing number of senators and congressmen are backing legislation that would make it possible to introduce new drugs as soon as they prove to be safe instead of waiting to satisfy the FDA's criteria for effectiveness. This is a step in the right direction.

Listed below are some of the medical reports on which this article is based. They are available at medical schools and at many university libraries. If you decide to join the search for greater brainpower, these reports are a good place to begin. In reading them, please remember that "intelligence" is a complex system of data processing abilities and that the tests used in these papers measure only a few of them. Researchers often disagree over the effect of drugs on intelligence because they are testing different abilities or because the dosage of some drugs must be carefully tailored to each patient to achieve their desired effects.

REFERENCES

Agranoff. "Memory and Protein Synthesis." *Scientific American*, June (1967). Available as *Scientific American* Offprint, No. 1077.

Borison, et al. "Metabolisms of an Antidepressant Amino Acid." Anesthesiology Department, Mount Sinai Hospital, Chicago: 1978. Presented in poster session at the April 9-14, 1978, meeting of the Federation of American Societies for Experimental Biology, Atlantic City, N.J.

Bylinsky. *Mood Control*, New York: Scribner's, 1978.

Drachman and Leavitt "Human Memory and the Cholinergic System." *Archives of Neurology*, 30 (1974): 113.

Enesco. "Effect of Vitamin B_{12} on Neuronal RNA and on Instrumental Conditioning in the Rat." *Recent Advances in Biological Psychiatry*, Vol. X (1968): Ch. 11.

Ferris, et al. "Senile Dementia: Treatment with Deanol." *Journal of the American Geriatrics Society*, June (1977): 241-44.

Goodman and Gilman. *The Pharmacological Basis of Therapeutics*, 4th ed. new York: Macmillan, 1970. See Ch. 40: Vasopressin and Oxytocin.

Hirsh and Wurtman. "Lecithin Consumption Increases Acetylcholine Concentrations in Rat Brain and Adrenal Gland." *Science*, 202 (1978): 223-25.

Hochschild. "Effect of Dimethylaminoethanol on the Lifespan of Senile Male A/J Mice." *Experiments in Gerontology*, 8 (1973): 185-91.

Landfield. "Computer-Determined EEG Patterns Associated with Memory-Facilitating Drugs and with ECS." *Brain Research Bulletin*, 1 (1976): 9-17.

Legros, et al. "Influence of Vasopressin on Memory and Learning." *The Lancet*, 7 January (1978): 41.

Nandy and Bourne. "Effect of Centrophenoxine (dimethlaminoethanol *p*-chlorophenoxyacetate) on the Lipofuscin Pigments in the Neurons of Senile Guinea Pigs." *Nature* (London), 210 (1966): 313-14.

Nathanson and Greengard. "Second Messengers in the Brain." *Scientific American*, August (1977): 108-19. Available as *Scientific American* Offprint, No. 1368.

Oliveros, et al. "Vasopressin in Amnesia." *The Lancet*, 7 January (1978): 42.

Peltzman. "Regulation of Pharmaceutical Innovation," *The Effects of the 1962 Kefauver Amendments on Introduction of New Drugs in the U.S.* American Enterprise Institute for Public Policy Research. Washington, D. C.: 1974.

Physician's Desk Reference. Oradell, N. J.: Medical Economics Co.

"RNA and the Memory," Brody, et al., eds. *Aging*. Vol. 1: *Clinical, Morphologic, and Neurochemical Aspects in the Aging Central Nervous System*. pp. 153-55. New York: Raven Press, 1975.

Seiden and Dykstra, *Psychopharmacology— A Biochemical and Behavioral Approach*, New York: Van Nostrand-Reinhold, 1977.

Sitaram, et al. "Human Serial Learning: Enhancement with Arecoline and Choline and Impairment with Scopolamine Correlate with Performance on Placebo." *Science*, 201 (1978): 274-76.

"Workshop on Advances in Experimental Pharmacology of Hydergine." *Gerontology*, 24 (1978). Suppl. 1: 1-154.

ORTHOHEALING

By Belinda Dumont

Clannng! The alarm clock's nerve-shattering jangle goads you into a groggy wakefulness that makes you feel as if you'd never slept. Nausea stirs your innards, and your mouth tastes as if the Russian army had tramped through with their boots on. Your body is telling you it needs help. At the doctor's office, they collect the standard urine and blood samples. Then a nurse clips a two-inch lock from your back hairline with thinning shears. "Not to disturb the hairdo," she says with a smile. You try not to glower.

The doctor checks your tongue, then your fingernails. He asks about past illnesses, examines you, and fills out a detailed chart of your exercise and eating habits. "I'll run this on the computer," he says briskly, then goes out.

He returns with the report in a few minutes. "The stress you've been under has raised your nutrient requirements," he announces. "You're seriously low on zinc, magnesium, and B vitamins, and you're way over on lead. It's a good thing you came in now. I'd hate to get you after your depression got worse and someone put you on tranks or mood elevators."

The prescription is downright strange: his own vitamin formula, a mineral preparation, large doses of vitamin C, and "eat eggs and applesauce once a day. We have to get that lead chelated. And no coffee. You might try pumpkin seeds for the zinc; that acne is a zinc deficiency. Your zinc and B-vitamin deficiencies account for the bad skin and irritability. But the most important thing is to check for lead sources at work.

"Get plenty of rest, exercise, and sunshine," he adds, then laughs. "That's a cliche, isn't it?"

Doctors who believe in it define orthomolecular medicine as the practice of maintaining good health by making certain all our nutritional needs are met and of treating disease by manipulating the natural body chemistry. Orthomolecular physicians give drugs when they must, but they try to avoid them. Instead, they work to strengthen the body's defenses, often using vitamins, minerals, and other nutrients.

"Disease in most cases is a chemical imbalance, inborn or induced, and nutrition is chemistry," said Dr. Michael Lesser, a founder of the Society of Orthomolecular Medicine. "We don't say drugs and surgery are bad, just that the physician should first try to correct the problem nutritionally."

Orthomolecular therapy may be the medicine

of the future, a low-technology alternative to today's mass-production health care. Though orthomolecular doctors remain the center of one of medicine's most heated controversies, they are attracting patients in growing numbers. ("I have to keep getting new patients," Dr. Lesser notes. "My old ones keep getting well so fast.") Other physicians are grudgingly beginning to accept their findings:

• Antibiotics work better when you take two grams of vitamin C with each dose.

• Some babies need so much vitamin B_6 that only massive injections will prevent continual convulsions. Most doctors would have said large vitamin supplements were needed only to cure such long-term deficiency diseases as scurvy and pellagra.

• Fully 10 percent of the diagnosed "crazies" in some Deep South mental hospitals were really suffering from a niacin deficiency brought on by their high-corn diet. When they were given the vitamin, the symptoms cleared and they were released.

• Lead poisoning sharply cuts IQ and efficiency, even at lead concentrations too low to show up in blood tests—levels physicians thought harmless. In children, they have found it by testing baby teeth.

• Cabbage, Brussels sprouts, and broccoli contain cancer-preventing chemicals, according to biochemists Elizabeth and James Miller, of the University of Wisconsin. Steve Tannenbaum, of MIT, adds vitamin C and alpha-tocopherol, a form of vitamin E, to the list. And Dr. Paul Mc-

Cay, of the Oklahoma Medical Research Foundation, says that a vitamin-A derivative called 13-cis-retinoic acid seems to combat cancers of the bladder, breast, colon, esophagus, lungs, and pancreas.

Such reports come as no surprise to people who have been trying to keep themselves healthy through good nutrition ever since Adelle Davis assembled all the research she could find into the popular book *Let's Eat Right to Keep Fit,* first published in 1954. "Adelle was the founder," acknowledges Dr. Robert Cathcart III, an osteopath who practices in Incline Village, Nevada, and a pioneer in the clinical use of vitamins. "Orthomolecular medicine has advanced far past her," he adds.

Davis's point was that our bodies must always get enough of the 40-odd nutrients they can't synthesize, particularly when we are under stress. If anything is missing, we become sick. Illness, she believed, is clear proof that something has been wrong with our diet. And she thought that food, especially vitamins and minerals, could treat disease, not just help us avoid it.

Modern nutritional therapy got its start in 1949, when Dr. Fred Klenner, chief of staff at Memorial Hospital, Reidsville, North Carolina, told of successfully treating viral diseases, including polio, with enormous doses of vitamin C — up to 100 grams a day given intravenously.

Several years later two Canadian psychiatrists tested a nutritional therapy for schizophrenia. Drs. Abraham Hoffer and Humphrey Osmond reported that the then-standard treatments — psychotherapy and electric shock — were 80-percent more effective when backed up by a high-protein, low-carbohydrate diet, with megadoses of niacin, nicotinic acid, B vitamins, and vitamin C.

Chemist Linus Pauling finally coined the term *orthomolecular medicine* in 1968: from *orthos,* Greek for "corrective," and *molecular,* for the body's chemical makeup. Nutritionists, a few open-minded doctors and medical researchers, and outright health nuts rallied round it.

But the infant field lacked crucial data: No one really knew what the normal human body needs to remain healthy. Finally, Dr. Roger Williams, director of the Clayton Foundation Biochemical Institute at the University of Texas, in Austin, worked out a basic list, which he called a "vitamin and mineral formulation for nutritional insurance." Most orthomolecular doctors still use his estimates in preference to the recommended daily allowances published by the National Research Council.

Unlike many orthomolecular theorists, Dr. Williams had plenty of professional prestige. He had discovered pantothenic acid (a B vitamin found in all living tissue, especially the liver, and essential for metabolism and hormone synthesis), and he was a member of the National Academy of Sciences. He developed the idea that people are as different in biochemistry as they are in appearance, and he put science behind the orthomolecular practice of tailoring the diet to the individual. In a less controversial field, his backing might have won respectability for the new approach.

Yet today its adherents remain a small band of hardy pioneers, for obvious reasons. They hold beliefs and practice medical rites that seem as strange to traditional physicians as the early Mormons seemed to devout nineteenth-century Protestants. Many are not even physicians. Nurses, biochemists, psychologists, even drug-rehabilitation workers and parole officers have been practicing orthomolecular methods. Many of them live in California, where the nuts come from. It hasn't helped their cause.

By implication, and sometimes openly, orthomolecular physicians stand as a reproach to the rest of medicine. Other doctors believe hypoglycemia, periodic weakness due to low blood sugar, is rare. Orthomolecular doctors think it's common, just not properly diagnosed. Orthomolecular physicians think that such pollutants as lead, mercury, and cadmium are common causes of illness, and they routinely test hair samples for evidence of poisoning. Others do not. If orthomolecular physicians are correct, other doctors are not fully doing their job.

The idea that disease can be treated by diet is one of the oldest in medicine. "The ancients were all nutritionists," the Orthomolecular Society's Dr. Lesser observes. "Hippocrates, the father of medicine, twenty-five hundred years ago said, 'Let thy food be thy medicine, and thy medicine be thy food.' Maimonides, in the thirteenth century, said, 'Let nothing that can be treated by diet be treated by any other means.'"

But modern men of medicine haven't been much impressed by this philosophy. A spokesman for the American Medical Association says only that "we haven't seen any sign that [orthomolecular medicine] works. Nutrition is by no means something that the medical profession ignores. We just take a rather conservative view."

The medical establishment's response to the use of vitamins in treating schizophrenia by Drs. Hoffer and Osmond was fairly typical: There almost wasn't any. The report coincided with the introduction of tranquilizers to treat schizophrenia, and it was drowned out by excitement over the wonder drugs.

Medicine's habit of resorting to drugs distresses some orthomolecular physicians, who are certain they have found a better way to treat their patients. It angers others.

"The neuroleptics [major tranquilizers] allowed for more humane control and speedier discharge," Dr. Lesser, who trained in orthodox psychiatry at Albert Einstein College of Medicine, in New York, admits. "But the side effects are so serious that people stop taking them and land back in the hospital. We wound up with swinging-door psychiatry."

Dr. Bernard Rimland, a San Diego pediatrician, is harsher in his criticism. "Modern medicine is bankrupt," he declares. "It's becoming a nightmare. The advances have often backfired, leaving in their wake death, blindness, stroke, and a variety of other iatrogenic [physician-caused] disasters more serious than the original disease. The side effects of prescription drugs now equal breast cancer as a leading cause of death in the United States.

"The difference between a schizophrenic and a normal person is not that the schizophrenic has a deficiency of Thorazine. The difference between a hyperactive kid and a normal one is not that the hyperactive kid has a deficiency of amphetamine or Ritalin. That's not a rational approach."

Traditional medicine's counterattacks on orthomolecular theorists are more organized and — among scientists — just as telling. Orthomolecular physicians don't do proper research, they charge. "What they do varies so widely that we can't exactly study it," the AMA says.

In 1973 the American Psychiatry Association's Task Force on Vitamin Therapy in Psychiatry told of repeating the studies that orthomolecular physicians feel prove that vitamins can help cure schizophrenia and other mental illnesses. They couldn't get the same results that orthomolecular researchers claimed. In medicine that's tantamount to saying the treatment doesn't work.

According to Dr. Lesser, though, the test says more about the way orthodox medicine does things than about orthomolecular practices. "They varied only one nutrient at a time, for example, administering niacin without a low-carbohydrate diet," he testified before the Senate's Select Committee on Nutrition and Human Needs. "It's the classic way drugs are tested in medicine, but it's oversimplified."

Dr. Hoffer, the pioneering schizophrenia researcher, adds that "their method is suitable for testing individual drugs, but it is virtually impossible to test a complex treatment method with it.

We change the treatment for each individual, and the dosage must sometimes be chosen by trial and error, as we do with diabetes. It's impossible to arrive at the correct dosage in their double-blind studies, in which the physician observing the results doesn't know what a given patient is receiving."

Yet most orthomolecular treatments are based on careful scientific research. Dr. Rimland himself provides a good example of how it gets done. Autistic children suffer a purely emotional illness, according to traditional medicine, but psychotherapy has proved heartbreakingly unsuccessful. Rimland has found an orthomolecular treatment that apparently works.

Like many orthomolecular researchers Rimland got into the field "anecdotally"—because he had seen a specific case. "I have an autistic son," he explains. "I began hearing from parents who tried what Adelle Davis suggested and found that it helped."

To aid in his research, Rimland called in two scientists with solid establishment credentials. One, psychiatrist Enoch Callaway, of the Langley Porter Neuropsychiatric Institute, in San Francisco, joined in because he thought "orthomolecular psychologists tend to do poor research and engage in polemics."

Rimland and his colleagues' study was eventually published in the prestigious *American Journal of Psychiatry*. Although orthodox psychiatrists claim that autistic children suffer an emotional illness, the researchers found that some, not all, are helped by massive doses of vitamin B_6, combined with a special diet and vitamin C. Rimland now runs the Institute for Child Behavior Research, in San Diego, to continue the work.

It seems, though, that not even careful research can win acceptance for some orthomolecular methods. The use of vitamin C in colds is so hotly contested that not even its startling endorsement by Dr. Pauling, in his book *Vitamin C and the Common Cold*, published ten years ago, could make it respectable. On the contrary, it evoked mutterings that the two-time Nobel Prize winner had finally gone senile.

Several careful medical trials of vitamin C have been performed since then, and the furor still hasn't abated. A recent editorial in *The Lancet,* one of England's leading medical journals, declared that vitamin C does not cut the number of colds people get, but it conceded that patients who used it had milder symptoms than others.

Dr. Pauling is still working with vitamin C, testing it now as an aid to cancer therapy. He and Dr. Ewan Cameron find that terminal-cancer patients, if given huge doses of ascorbic acid, live about three times as long as they otherwise would. Yet he reports that "we've applied to the National Cancer Institute five times for a grant. We do it once a year, at least. So far they've said no. It's a little hard to satisfy them. We'd have to withhold the therapy from half our patients."

Orthomolecular doctors are finding a wide variety of other uses for vitamin C. Nevada's Dr. Cathcart treats about 1,000 new patients a year in his Incline Village practice and reports that "massive doses of C ease viral infections. In the nine years that I've been in Incline Village, which has a generally young population, we've never hospitalized a patient for viral disease."

In fact, Cathcart classifies illnesses by how much ascorbic acid it takes to cure them. "Hepatitis is a sixty-gram disease," he says. "The hippies here all know how to treat it. They come down out of the hills, buy their little can of vitamin C powder, and cure it for about seven dollars."

Patients take vitamin C up to "bowel tolerance"—until they develop diarrhea. "Colds are a hundred-gram disease," Cathcart says. "When they hit, people can take eight grams without diarrhea. They know they've got something, but ninety percent of the symptoms are blocked."

Scientific studies haven't confirmed vitamin C's effectiveness, he believes, because the experimenters used too little of it. The largest dose used in double-blind studies so far is four grams a day. "Everyone's different," Cathcart stresses. "You have to take each patient right up to bowel tolerance."

There is a darker side to vitamin C, however. "People become dependent on ascorbic," Cathcart asserts. "These are people on a high-maintenance dose, say, over four grams a day. Hay fever sufferers, for example, take ten or fifteen grams a day for years. When you take it, there's a sudden punch, and you feel better."

He warns that if someone using large doses of vitamin C is suddenly deprived of it, say, when hospitalized after an accident, it can be dangerous. "They'll do very badly," he says. "We're getting to the point where it will be malpractice to take away someone's vitamin C."

As the battle over ascorbic acid continues, several other battles are shaping up. One of the most bitter is being fought against the Food and Drug Administration, long an enemy of unorthodox new therapies. Orthomolecular methods are a thorn in the FDA's side, because the agency cannot regulate the use of vitamins and other natural substances as it does artificial drugs. Recently the FDA has attacked experimentation with adrenal cortical extract (ACE).

Patients deficient in adrenal hormones develop fatigue and put on excess weight, particularly around the hips. Doctors usually give them synthetic steroids, with dangerous side effects. Dr. Richard P. Heumer, of Westlake Village, California, insists that ACE injections are as effective as steroids and free of the hazards. He gives them along with nutritional therapy and B vitamins, especially B_6, and can often wean patients away from other drugs.

Unfortunately, the FDA has classified ACE as a "new drug." This classification makes ACE difficult to obtain, even for research. "Their first commandment is 'Thou shalt not experiment with substances naturally occurring in the human body,'" Cathcart says bitterly. Though the FDA remains unmoved by calls for controlled studies of ACE, Senator Barry Goldwater has thrown his support behind the orthomolecular researchers, calling the report that led to the ban "peculiar and scanty." Whether Goldwater's backing will do any good remains to be seen.

Orthomolecular research has also focused on the sex hormones. Estrogens, for example, are often given for toxemia or bleeding in the first months of pregnancy. According to Dr. Ray Peat, a research chemists, they can combine with unsaturated fats in the diet, causing the birth of small-brained, retarded animals. He claims that using 10 to 15 grams of the hormone progesterone, instead of estrogens, during pregnancy raises a child's IQ by around 35 points. And even the AMA says that progesterone is harmless to both fetus and mother when given in early pregnancy.

Dr. Peat blames excess estrogen for many ills: "There is an epidemic of prolactin-secreting pituitary tumors," he asserts. "They are the result of the Pill, which contains large doses of estrogen. Progesterone stops it." Other maladies, he says, may be caused by progesterone deficiency. Among them are conditions that mimic epilepsy, multiple sclerosis, and, surprisingly, estrogen deficiency. All these conditions can be treated effectively with a progesterone skin cream, Peat reports.

We'll soon be adding antioxidants to our morning's dose of vitamins and minerals if orthomolecular physicians have their way. Antioxidants prevent oxygen, and some other elements, from attacking easily damaged body molecules. Many of the chemicals in air pollution are oxidants. Vitamins A, C, and E are the best-known antioxidants, but some of the trace minerals are also effective.

Two possible antioxidants that have gained attention recently are zinc and selenium. "We think selenium will be to the Eighties what iodine was to the early 1900s," says Herb Boynton, president of a La Jolla, California, health-food business called Nutrition 21. "We're just beginning to find out that most Americans are deficient in it." The company regularly searches the scientific literature for new nutritional findings and offers to answer queries about human dietary requirements.

It begins to look as if orthomolecular doctors are slowly convincing their more conservative colleagues. Dr. Hossein Ghadimi, a Long Island pediatrician, for instance, is a specialist in metabolic diseases who says he doesn't think orthomolecular medicine is even a legitimate specialty. Yet he gives vitamin C to make antibiotics more effective, uses amino acids and megavitamin therapy, and tests diabetics and hypoglycemics even more rigorously than most orthomolecular practitioners would.

He explains that "there are biochemical reasons to use vitamins in far greater dosages than is done in conventional medicine, which says that if you don't feel right, it's part of aging and that you can take Valium to lift your mood. I believe we can manipulate you nutritionally so that, with no drugs, no stimulants, you can start to feel like a new person."

Modern medicine, he agrees, pays far too little attention to nutrition. "Cancer patients often die from malnutrition," he charges. " 'Overwhelming infection' kills them. No wonder they can't fight off even a little infection. All they're given is a five-percent glucose solution.

"One of the richest men in the world died of starvation. Aristotle Onassis had myasthenia gravis and couldn't chew. Just like those patients under conventional therapy in intensive-care units, they gave him intravenous glucose. Patients on such a miserable diet die from malnutrition. They should have given him amino acids."

There is a lot of nutritional research, Dr. Ghadimi said. "Doctors know it, but the research doesn't cross over. It just hasn't been used at the bedside."

At long last, that may be changing. Only ten or so medical schools have separate departments to teach nutrition—"and they're lousy," Dr. Lesser said—but the number is slowly increasing. Perhaps the orthomolecular doctors have finally made their point.

There is little doubt that the health nuts were right all along, especially about preventive medicine. Our nutritional needs are more individualized and far more critical to our health than traditionalists have thought.

Though our needs vary and critics claim that orthomolecular practices vary even more, Dr. Lesser points out that there are some basic principles of good health that nearly all the orthomolecular physicians adhere to. It couldn't hurt to include them in our own diets.

"Lesser is more," the psychiatrist quips. "Eat unprocessed foods as much as possible, trying for organically grown fruits and vegetables. Avoid frozen foods. They are treated with chelating agents—the wrong kind. No canned foods. They are contaminated with sugar and salt. Avoid processed and refined foods. No white flour. No sugar. Use maple sugar or unfiltered honey if you like sweeteners. Avoid coffee, alcohol, and the city. If you can't, you may have to supplement your basic diet."

He recommends "B vitamins in as balanced a form as possible, such as brewer's yeast." For vitamin E, his rule of thumb is to take 100 units per day for each decade of your life. Vitamins A and D should be taken in a ten-to-one ratio, say, 25,000 units of A and 2,500 of D daily, as Adelle Davis prescribed. Add a natural mineral preparation that has as many elements as possible.

Scientists still haven't figured out for certain how much vitamin C healthy people need. Estimates of the proper daily dose range from 100 milligrams up to Dr. Cathcart's four grams per day. Whatever you take, you'll need more when you're ill or under stress. There is some evidence that you should also take more of vitamins A and D and minerals, especially calcium.

"Pay attention to everything you consume," Lesser urges. "You can't expect to be healthy if you put toxins in your body. If you are really ill, see a physician. The best of them understand nutrition."

For further information on nutrition and orthomolecular medicine, contact the Orthomolecular Medical Society, 2340 Parker Street, Berkeley, California 94704.

DR. C.'S VITAMIN ELIXIRS

By Kathleen Stein

For demonstration purposes, Dr. Michael Colgan has offered us his body. The New Zealand scientist, currently a visiting scholar at Rockefeller University, in New York City, says his individualized vitamin-and-mineral program is now sufficiently developed to permit people to carry out strenuous activities over a period of weeks "on nothing but a handful of pills — and water. And get stronger in the process."

Colgan would be happy to prove it by spending a week or ten days in the Adirondacks with his vitamins, "hiking over one of the really hard trails through the mountains." He suggests a group of scientists might try to keep up with him. He would, of course, be fitted out in astronaut fashion with a modified Resperonics microchip cardiac-monitoring device to telemeter continuous readouts of his heart rate, blood pressure, and other vital signs to a remote recorder. There is no doubt in Colgan's mind that he would come back fitter than when he left. But, then, the forty-three-year-old nutritionist ran the 1981 New York Marathon in four hours only five weeks after he suffered a debilitating torn leg muscle — and with no intervening training.

We tend to believe Colgan about the Adirondacks experiment. If he steals a week away from his research, he'll probably do it. At one time, however, we were more skeptical. That's before we came to realize that the history of nutrition in twentieth-century industrialized society reads like a black-humor atrocity tale in which the more we overeat, the less nourishment we get; in which people are actually starving to death as they wallow in fat. And that was also before we ourselves were suited into Dr. Colgan's biochemically customized vitamin and mineral supplements and began to feel intimations of Amazonian strengths.

Colgan is one of a rapidly growing group of scientists who are attempting to refine nutrition into an exact science. Colgan thinks it is an absolutely necessary thing to do. "Western man," he says, "is in danger of losing the use of his legs. He doesn't get enough exercise, eats a great deal of food with little nutritive value, and ingests a large number of toxins into his system." Since World War II — and the invention of K rations — peoples of the "developed" countries have undergone a huge dietary revolution. In 35 years a small-town, single-farmer growing-and-marketing network has mutated into a monolithic, highly integrated infrastructure in which, says Ross Hume Hall, in

Food for Naught, "the object is not to nourish, or even to feed, but to force an ever-increasing consumption of fabricated products." Until recently this transformation has gone unmarked by government agencies and learned bodies alike. It has not, however, gone totally unnoticed by the supermarket-going public, who in expanding numbers are getting worried that they are indeed becoming what they eat.

When people ask Colgan why, with all the advances in modern medicine, they need to take extra vitamins and minerals, he tells them that modern medicine is not making them healthier or live longer. Colgan will cite many findings, the most compelling of which is probably *The Impact of Nutrition on the Health of Americans*, by eminent pediatrician and public-health scientist Joseph Beasley, Bard Fellow in Medicine and Nutrition at Bard College, Annandale-on-Hudson, New York. In this report, in final preparation for the Ford Foundation, Beasley presents evidence that resoundingly contradicts the government's claim that Americans have never been healthier. "In stark contrast to the picture painted by the Surgeon General," Beasley says, "some illnesses, symptoms, and conditions are rising markedly — degenerative diseases that afflict upward of 100 million Americans." The plague list is long and includes everything from massive killers like cancer and cardiovascular diseases, to diabetes, arthritis, birth defects, retardation, obesity, hypoglycemia, alcoholism, mental illnesses, drug addiction, and legions of more chronic afflictions. Beasley designates this burgeoning phenomenon the Malnutrition-Poisoning Syndrome. And, he says, our traditional medical methodology is faltering in the face of these chronic degenerative diseases, because "it is unduly narrow in focus, too inflexible and restricted in its considerations of causes and connections."

To help turn the tide of this "epidemic," Colgan calls for a new order — "to turn the face of medicine away from disease toward health, toward preventive medicine, toward individual biochemistry, which is just the opposite of mass medicine, which is just not working anymore." Colgan predicts that within 25 years there will be a significant shift toward custom-tailored health care, which will involve "relatively simple manipulations a person can do to maintain his own body."

Colgan views his own vitamin-and-mineral supplement program as such a simple manipulation. The correct daily dose of nutrient supplements can enhance physical and mental performance, fight pain and depression, and inhibit development of age degeneration in an individual and the diseases that are its inevitable result.

Although he dislikes being considered a "biological curiosity," Colgan is an excellent advertisement for his own system. He claims that before he developed his supplement program and started following it seven years ago, his rich chestnut hair was going gray and he got frequent colds and flu. "I guess I was of no more than average health: overweight, tired, and aging," he says. Today he has the sleek lines of an athlete and can run ten miles without effort. Ask him and he'll demonstrate a one-arm chin-up and then a one-arm push-up. "I always wanted to be able to do these things as a youth, but I never could. My strength has increased more than one hundred percent in the last seven years. And I've changed from a complete skeptic about vitamins to one completely convinced. When I began my work, my colleagues laughed. Now most of them take my formulas." Colgan hasn't had a cold in years, and his wife says he's impervious to "bugs." Perhaps only the expression in his luminous blue eyes gives a hint of the decades he's lived. At times they look as if they belong in another, older body.

The urgency of Colgan's mission—and it can be called that—is most clearly understood against the backdrop of nutritional statistics that dwarf our attempts to "eat right and stay healthy." Here's a small sampling (cited by Beasley, Colgan, and U.S. government sources):

• In both the United States and the United Kingdom the average life expectancy of an adult, twenty-five, has not changed for more than 30 years.

• In 1973 the Office of Technology Assessment (OTA) estimated that 70 percent of deaths were caused by diseases linked to diet, including high levels of fat, sugar, and salt.

• Autopsies of men between the ages of eighteen and twenty-two killed in World War I showed no signs of atherosclerosis, according to the *Journal of the American Medical Association*. In autopsies of American youths killed in Vietnam, it was rare to find a soldier who did not have athero-sclerotic disease.

• Since 1960 there has been a huge rise in the number of children with brain damage, hyperactivity, and learning disabilities. Today one child out of every five is afflicted.

• In 1910, 10 percent of U. S. food was factory-refined or treated with artificial additives. In 1981 almost 80 percent of our foods were processed.

• The amount of salt in frozen vegetables can be 100 percent more than in fresh vegetables.

• The use of food coloring increased 995 percent between 1940 and 1976.

• A "designer" fast-food meal—burger, milk shake, french fries—contains 22 chemical additives, 12 of which in fairly small amounts are known to be toxic.

• Fifty percent of an average American's total caloric intake comes in the form of "empty calories"—refined sugars and carbohydrates.

• An average American consumes nine pounds of additives annually.

• The OTA states conservatively that 30 percent of American men and 40 percent of the women between the ages of thirty and forty-nine are overweight. Twenty percent are by definition obese.

• The U.S. Recommended Daily Allowance (RDA) of vitamin A for pigs is 200 percent greater than it is for humans; for dogs, 300 percent greater.

• Two U. S. government studies found that 60 percent of those sampled who consumed a "good mixed diet," based on U. S. RDAs, showed clinical symptoms of malnutrition, regardless of income level.

• Because of the reduced need for chewing, refined foods lower the amount of saliva produced, and the entire metabolic processing and absorbing of nutrients are thereby reduced.

Our bodies, already being malnourished and progressively and simultaneously being poisoned, are treated to a catalog of additive insults. Beasley writes, "Every serving of processed food is treated with one or more dyes, bleaches, emulsifiers, antioxidants, moisturizers, desiccants, extenders, thickeners, disinfectants, defoliants, fungicides, neutralizers, artificial sweeteners, hydrolyzers, anticaking and antifoaming agents, curers, hydrogenators, fortifiers, antibiotics, arsenic, artificial sex hormones, and pesticides."

So it might seem that everyone in the Western World needs to be on a vitamin-mineral supplement program (not to mention the inhabitants of the Third World with their different and crisis-proportioned nutritional problems). Dr. Colgan, you may have come along just in time. Who would have thought the little molecules dubbed "vitamines" by Polish biochemist Casimir Funk—who discovered the first one, vitamin A, back in 1911—could be so vitally important? Today, together with the essential minerals, 48 various substances are recognized as absolutely requisite for full health. As long as one's diet supplies these nutrients, cells and tissues can synthesize the many thousands more compounds necessary for life.

An ultimate definition of vitamins has eluded science, although certain functional characteristics are shared by most vitamins. Vitamins are organic molecules essential for life—in man, beast, and plant—in minute quantities. Each vitamin performs a specific task that cannot be accomplished by any other substance. But, unlike their sister molecules—the hormones—vitamins (with few exceptions) cannot be made inside the body. They have to be imported in things that are eaten. The absence or diminution of a single vitamin causes biochemical disruptions.

In their catalytic role as coenzymes, vitamins assist enzymes and are critical to the growth, maintenance and repair of every cell. Because vitamins work synergistically—as a team—a single deficiency can threaten the cell's well-being. Vitamins also operate at large in the chemical processes of such tissues as the liver, brain, bone marrow, and kidneys, coordinating myriad bodily activities. The body cannot make use of what it eats without vitamins and minerals: although minerals, too, must be present in the body for it to sustain a biochemical balance, they are not chemically as fragile as vitamins, and they can be retained by the body much longer.

Colgan came to understand the importance of vitamins and minerals and discovered the fallacies of the good mixed diet via a strange route. Highways. Born in England, he studied civil engineering and traveled to New Zealand to build bridges and turnpikes. While on the design team of the Wellington Urban Motorway in 1967, he was struck by the idea that highways don't bring people together, but distance them. To find out why humans build highways, he returned to earn a doctorate in psychology at the University of Auckland. He was offered a lecturing position at the university and also was given the opportunity to administer a clinic at the University Medical School. It was there that he began his first nutritional analyses. "A very smart M. D. was there," Colgan remembers, "who kept saying, 'These people coming in with earaches, stomachaches, joint pain, depression — the trouble with them is they're undernourished.' It was just a general comment, but I thought about it."

Colgan and his colleagues researched the nutritional literature and drew up a chart of malnourishment symptoms, which they put on a wall. Whenever a patient showed any of the symptoms, the clinicians noted them. "We suddenly realized that almost everyone coming to the clinic was malnourished," he says. "As far as we could determine, however, they all ate reasonably good diets." Colgan began analyzing their food, and he was stunned. It contained nothing like the amounts of nutrients given in the nutritional tables. Some oranges, for example, contained no vitamin C at all. "The tables were sheer nonsense," he recalls. (Today Colgan points out that the American Medical Association has for 15 years recognized that the nutrient content of fresh foods can vary enormously, depending on soil, weather, and the time of harvesting, and can fall to zero during some methods of processing.)

Since the good mixed diet wasn't doing the job, Colgan decided to give his patients carefully controlled supplements. But before handing them out, he began analyzing the vitamin pills and, to his consternation, found they were not true to label. "It was a real can of worms. Single nutrients did not contain stated amounts, and multivitamin-mineral formulations did not follow prescribed mixtures of quantities." (Of the brands tested, Colgan found only Parke-Davis and Healtheries, Ltd., contained what they claimed to contain.) "In some cases," he says, "the formula appeared to reflect more the commercial advantages of being able to put everything in one pill, including negligible quantities of expensive substances, instead of the requirements of human nutrition."

But what about the requirements? Colgan's next can of worms was dosage. How much and in what combinations? "Initially physicians associated with our group contended we should provide a supplement conforming to the U.S. or British RDAs. But after conducting analyses of these RDAs, we decided they were inadequate." The premise upon which RDAs have been established is "an absence of disease." But Colgan cautions that minimizing disease is a far cry from maximizing health.

Since little research has been conducted in assessing the optimum RDAs in humans, Colgan has been forced to turn to veterinary medicine. The assessment of supplementation levels in the breeding of livestock is now a considerable science. Thoroughbred horses, as well as pedigree cats and dogs, are better fed than their owners, he says. In view of livestock nutrient tables, Colgan began mapping out a set of criteria for determining quantity and combinations that human individuals should have, and means for determining whether or not the dosage was producing the right effect. He compiled a list of 231 variables related to biochemical, clinical, and behavioral evidence of deficiency levels. "Nature best responds to a logically and carefully thought out questionnaire," Colgan quotes from the eminent scientist Sir Ronald Fisher. And he developed one with detailed queries about an individual's health and eating, social, and emotional habits. Included for evaluation are biochemical analyses of the subject's hair, fingernails, and blood.

The most difficult consideration was the synergistic nature of nutrient interactions. Although this holistic nature of nutrients is of primary importance in achieving maximum health, most research has been conducted on single nutrients in ways that do not permit the synergy to occur. "The researcher," says Beasley, "who attempts to study the impact of a single nutrient, such as vitamin C or E or zinc, without regard to the complexity of human chemical processes is betrayed by the standard methodology itself."

"It took the human body at least three million years to evolve," Colgan notes. "During that time the organism learned to use synergistically a large number of substances. When Nature put it all together, she wasn't considering the ways scientists would come to classify chemicals, but was taking the whole mix available amd making the organism fit it as best it could.

"Today, especially with our internal and external pollution," he continues, "an understanding of multiple nutrient interactions and their interaction with toxins is essential. Most physicians, as well as lay people, are ignorant of these complex processes, and most vitamin-mineral supplements are gulped down haphazardly, sometimes by the fistful, with only the flimsiest reasoning — or no reasoning at all — behind the self-dosing or doctor's prescription. The biochemical individuality of each person indicates that most commercial formulas are unlikely to work, no matter how 'super,' 'mega,' or 'multi' the label.

"Also, the varying environmental conditions to which each person is exposed radically alter his supplement needs. A man who smokes twenty cigarettes a day, for example, is under constant biochemical stress and may require fifteen times the RDA of vitamin C to avoid suppression of immune-system function. Women taking oral contraceptives may require as much as ten times the RDA of vitamin B-twelve, six times the RDA of vitamin B-six, and four times the RDA of folic acid to maintain normal cardiovascular function and lipid metabolism."

In 1973 Colgan began giving personalized supplementation to patients; since then he has treated more than 1,000 people, always developing and refining his methodology. From the earliest case studies the results were telling. His New Zealand subjects on whom he has complete data include 11 obese females, 3 female and 6 male alcoholics, 16 female depressives, 9 female and 3 male schizophrenics, 9 hyperactive children, and many others suffering from various paranoias, anxiety reactions, asthma, hypertension — and 74 athletes. "We've had incredible changes in people," Colgan says, and he rates his successes at about 75 percent.

Certain cases sound like miracle cures: There was the malnourished woman on antidepressants who binged on junk food when she was depressed and thereby aggravated her malnourishment. After three months on her supplements she lost 15 pounds. Her heart rate and blood pressure dropped; her blood sugar stabilized. After six months she was no longer depressed and was weaned from the antidepressants.

And there was the case of one elderly woman amost incapacitated by chronic osteoarthritis. On Colgan's vitamin-mineral dosage her arthritis gradually improved to the point where she could go shopping with friends. Previously she had not left home in several years.

But Colgan's prize case is a maximum-security-prison convict with a 12-year history of psychosis, violent crime, uncontrollable rage, disorientation, and schizophrenic symptoms. He was somewhat obese, lacking in energy, a junk-food addict. Today, after nine years on supplementation, Colgan reports, he has no recurrence of the mental problems. His whole temperament has changed. When the fellow was released from prison, Colgan helped him get accepted to the University of Auckland, where he finished a double degree in 1980. "Now he's slim and strong," Colgan says. "He's become the kindest, gentlest person I know."

Although this anecdotal evidence has its own

rewards, Colgan was having trouble collecting hard data for nutritional studies. The patients' manifold clinical problems were confounding the purely nutritional information. Colgan chose to test the healthiest people he could find — athletes. And to date, perhaps the most reliable information on human nutrient supplementation comes from his pilot studies with two polarities of athletic performers: long-distance runners and weight lifters. Could any of these men, already in good shape and eating a reasonably well balanced diet, be transformed into a Hercules or Achilles by changing his nutrition?

In a double-blind experiment with ten experienced marathon runners aged twenty-eight to forty-four, five runners supplemented with Colgan's nutrients for six months bettered their marathon times by an average of 17 minutes and 44 seconds. One thirty-eight-year-old sliced his time from two hours 59 minutes to 2:30. A forty-year-old shaved his record from 2:48 to 2:33. Runners given the placebo bettered their times by an average of six minutes and 43 seconds. (Throughout 1982 Colgan is conducting a year-long study of 40 marathoners at Rockefeller University, many of whom ran in the 1981 New York Marathon. It will be interesting to see whether they beat Alberto Salazar this year.)

The weight-lifters experiment examined the effects of nutrients on an extremely different physical performance. Four experienced iron pumpers, matched for age, lifting ability, and stage of training, were divided into two groups. Colgan devised two strength tests: a slantbroad biceps curl with dumbbells and a slantboard leg raise with weights. In addition, he measured performance at the Olympic lifts — press and clean and jerk. This experiment, also a double blind, was more complicated. Colgan switched supplements to placebo after three months for one group and changed placebo to supplements in the other group. The results after six months demonstrated a 50 percent increase in the strength tests after three months on the vitamin-mineral regimen. The lifters who started out on the supplements showed the 50 percent increase during the first three months, followed by a discernible slump during the period on placebo. For the musclemen who began with the placebo, the second half of the period was a time of dramatic improvement in their strength. In the Olympic lifts, the supplemented periods showed a 6 percent gain compared to a less than 1 percent gain in the unsupplemented periods. A 6 percent increase in poundage pressed is enough to elevate a lifter from ignominy to a gold medal. And Colgan reminds us that these were men near the limits of their strength before the study began. They had all used nutrient supplements for years on what Colgan called an "ad libitum" regimen.

Besides the obvious performance changes, beneficial physiological changes were occurring in these athletes' bodies. For the runners there were small but reliable reductions in heart rate, blood pressure, cholesterol level, and triglycerides (fats) in all subjects, and increased hemoglobin in two. There was evidence the supplemented runners had fewer minor injuries and infections and missed fewer days in training. "These data suggest," Colgan says, "that supplementation exerted a positive effect upon the immune system. These data are in accord with growing evidence of immune-system enhancement by vitamin-mineral supplementation."

In clinic patients, runners and weight lifters alike, Colgan saw unexpected results. In all groups there was improved hair, skin, and fingernail condition. There was a lessening of longstanding complaints, including susceptibility to infection, herpes simplex, acne, eczema, chronic joint, muscle, land back pains, constipation, nervous indigestion, headache, and sinusitis. There were reports of improved memory and alertness. Colgan noticed that all these conditions were more marked in older subjects. Further investigation led him to suspect that the supplements were having a general effect and might be reducing some of the degenerative symptoms of aging. So he conducted a longevity study with 12 rats from weaning until death — 6 on supplemented chow, 6 not. The rodents on supplements lived 24 percent longer than the control rats and enjoyed healthier lives.

Are there any indications of rejuvenatory effects in Colgan's vitamin-mineral supplement in someone middle-aged or older? "There is absolutely no doubt anymore," he replies. "For example, it has been confirmed by a number of laboratories now that atherosclerosis can be reversed by dietary changes. Atherosclerosis is one of the major degenerative diseases and affects almost everyone by middle age. If you can remove plaque from inside the arteries, restore the arterial wall, reabsorb scar tissue, you are really reversing aging." Colgan speculates that within the next 25 years human life expectancy can be increased considerably. "But it's not going to come from curative medicine or replacement of organs and glands. It's going to come from repairing the system as it is.

"We must consider the human skin as constituting a giant test tube," he continues, 'a hairy bag filled with a mixture of chemicals. We can know what is going on inside each test tube by using computerized matrices to correlate the variables in the whole system. We can make changes in the test tube, put the right nutrients in it, and watch it develop without invading it. The body is such a dynamic system; every year or so it has a new shot at life. In that time there's a great turnover of cells. Even the liver can regenerate."

Not content to remain a spectator at this parade of living test tubes, this reporter volunteered to become a human bottle, a mobile statistic in Colgan's Health and Performance Nutrient Supplement Program. To become initiated, I donated hair for atomic-emission spectroscopic analysis (for mineral content), underwent a battery of blood tests to determine levels of cholesterol, triglycerides, glucose, red and white blood-cell count, hemoglobin, hematocrit, and other biochemical fractions. Blood pressure and heart rate were noted, as well as fingernail condition (nails are records of metabolic activity; even a two-day fast will leave its mark in the growing nail). Colgan's questionnaire is not as lengthy as it is targeted, with questions ranging from basic facts about one's body and its maintenance to queries about dream recall and emotional tone.

These questions were culled from many more by means of "item analysis," a mathematical technique. Items that yield correlations neither with physical conditions nor with other variables are discarded. An item such as the "sexual satisfaction scale" holds more of the variance than many others combined. "Excellent sexual functioning requires good health," Colgan says. "Any dysfunction will reduce sexual satisfaction; it's a delicate mechanism."

After the biochemical information was added to the questionnaire matrix, my equation was complete on one side. The other side was supplied by the 32 uniquely tailored nutrients I now take daily. And the effects? Within a few months I had clipped five minutes off my record for the one-mile freestyle, and without regular swimming workouts. I noticed a diminution of appetite, especially for junk food and other carbohydrates, including alcohol. A 1,200-mile mid-October sail in the Atlantic under ridiculously spartan conditions posed no energy crisis with Colgan's ubiquitous pill packets aboard. And the stresses of urban life seem to have receded. All this is of course anecdotal and not really admissible in scientific court. However, a sixth-month analysis of blood has generated tangible facts: blood pressure from 120/80 to 105/80 and cholesterol from 214 to 171 (milligrams per 100 milliliters of blood). "That could be a fairly significant drop," comments Dr. Daryl Isaacs, a specialist in internal medicine at New York's Beekman Hospital. "It augurs well for a modern American, although it's not as good as the ninety-five [mg/mls] you might find in the heart of Africa."

Like many former skeptics, I have become a zealous convert. I think everyone should be on a program such as Colgan's. But the big drawback is that such programs are not widely available, and when they are, they will be expensive ($1,000 for Colgan's). The goal of preventive medicine is such that people will be able to go to nutrition specialists as easily as they now go to dentists. Or the same way they drive their cars in for six-month tune-ups. That easy. Just 60 milligrams of para-amino-benzoic acid, please, and 50 units of mixed tocopherols. And check my triglycerides, if you don't mind.

Meantime, in the world of nutritional supplements, confusion reigns. In the front lines of the additive wars are the millions of Americans who are taking supplements. It has been stated that the 75 million Americans on supplements excrete the most expensive urine in the world, and indeed $2 billion was spent on nutritional components in 1980. And yet few people who take them know enough about what they're doing to effect any positive change. Ignorance is rampant. ("What I need is a big dose of vitamin G," is an example that was overheard in a restaurant recently.)

"Overdosing is the most common mistake," Colgan says. "People think that if they do well on thirty milligrams, well, why not six hundred? Part of my research is aimed at establishing a true level of efficiency so that people will not go out and buy a formula that's supermegamega, with five hundred milligrams of everything in it. That is just rubbish! It's a subclinical poisoning!"

Everyone's nutrient needs are different, but until such time as individual biochemistry clinics are in operation, Colgan has reluctantly offered a readily available combination of nutrients that should take the edge off one's deficiencies. "This daily formula is given against my better judgment," Colgan cautions, "but in hopes of doing more good than nothing."

Vitamin A (retinol)	15,000 IU
Vitamin B$_1$ (thiamine)	50 mg
Vitamin B$_2$ (riboflavine)	50 mg
Vitamin B$_3$ (niacin 25, niacinamide)	150 mg
Vitamin B$_5$ (pantothenic acid)	50 mg
Vitamin B$_6$ (pyridoxin)	75 mg
Vitamin B$_{12}$ (cyanocobalamin)	100 mcg
Folic acid	800 mcg
Biotin	600 mcg
Choline	125 mg
Inositol	125 mg
Para-aminobenzoic acid	100 mg
Vitamin C (ascorbic acid)	2,000 mg
Bioflavinoid complex	250 mg
Vitamin D (calciferol)	600 IU
Vitamin E (d-alpha-tocopherol)	400 IU
Pectin	50 mg
Calcium (Ca)	750 mg
Magnesium (Mg)	375 mg
Phosphorus (P)	400 mg
Potassium (K)	250 mg
Iron (Fe)	15 mg

Copper (Cu)	1 mg
Molybdenum (Mo)	75 mcg
Manganese (Mn)	10 mg
Zinc (Zn)	50 mg
Chromium (Cr) (glucose-tolerance factor)	125 mcg
Selenium (Se)	150 mcg
Nickel (Ni)	50 mcg
Vanadium (V)	50 mcg
Iodine (I)	200 mcg

(IU = International Units; mg = milligram; mcg = microgram)

Because of the proliferation of con artists in the health-food business, and the dangers of misuse of readily available supplements, scientists cannot make radical statements about nutrition to the public. Colgan gives the example of selenium: Ten states in the United States are deficient in this trace element, and these areas are associated with a threefold higher rise of heart disease because of this deficiency. "Yet one can't make a statement about selenium and heart disease," Colgan asserts, "because within one hour all the shops everywhere will be sold out of it. And there are lots of seleniums on the market, some quite useless, all highly toxic if taken in overdose."

And the food-processing industry? "Oh, they're interested in my work," Colgan smiles. "They offer me weekends, give me the stretch-limousine treatment. Actually, though, I'm more disillusioned by drug companies that make vitamins. Many are run by people who know nothing about nutrition, have not one qualified person on the executive staff. Or, if they have, these people spend all their time in other research and never come in contact with the vitamins that are being produced by the firm. There is so much rubbish on the market," he adds abruptly. "The majority of vitamins in health-food stores are rubbish!" After some thought, Colgan decided to endorse the Nature Plus range of commonly available vitamins as one brand he knows is true to label. "Let me add," he laughs, "that I do not own stock or have any commercial contract with that company. Merely, tests have shown that their supplements contain what they say they contain."

Best news for Colgan is the recent rise of interest in nutrition and preventive medicine. "We're not going to investigate it piecemeal, but in an integrated way. Historically that's the way it happened with biochemistry and molecular physics. The problems are far too complex for me to be working off in an isolated little lab." Colgan is collaborating with Rockefeller's Jay Weiss, a behavioral scientist whose 15-year research has yielded strong evidence that immunological function can decrease 50 percent under nonspecific stress. Colgan hopes to "tag on to" Weiss's experiments to find out whether nutrient supplements can decrease immunological damages caused by stress. "Nothing has ever been shown to protect you from stress," he explains; "none of the common medications, valium, nothing. If it can be demonstrated that a simple dietary maneuver can protect lymphocyte function, well," he grins, "that would support Linus Pauling's hypothesis and would certainly cause a bit of a stir in cancer research."

Colgan is completing a book on nutrition (to be published by Morrow this fall) and will open a clinic in Great Britain next year. It will accept all clients. It will provide nutritional supplementation for each according to his or her biochemical profile. "Taking into account," he says with a kind of Shakespearean flourish, "the strength with which the environment and oral gratification hold people to their pleasures, and the frailty of human willpower. The Colgan Program," he chuckles, "will correct for, as far as possible, the nutritional sins of the flesh. It took the last hundred years to invent means for humans to destroy their environments and themselves by internal and external pollutions. We need the most audacious, the most innovative developments in preventive medicine if this crisis is to be averted."

Colgan believes that if healthy people can keep away from toxic substances and achieve optimum nutrition, they can excel in any field to which they devote themselves. Limitless transformation. And since athletes are about the only people already intensely involved in this "experiment," Colgan turns again to them. "You can already see it in athletes," he says, "people like Sugar Ray Leonard. And Hearns. Or linebackers in football—if you compare them with linebackers twenty years ago, those people were still big, but they were big and fat, and could run fast maybe fifty yards. Today these guys are bigger still, but with muscle, and they are sprinting the hundred yards in eleven seconds. The same thing happened with the Olympics. You used to see people of all sizes and shapes competing. But now the athletes are like gladiators. It's due to our knowledge of nutrition and physiology. Every athlete I know takes vitamins. They say, 'I eat pasta, junk food, and so forth.' But what they don't say is, 'I have raw vegetables ground up in my blender every morning with my vitamins.' They don't say those things, because they don't want to give anybody the edge in top competition. It's very small, you know." Colgan on the other hand, wants to give everybody the edge. "It can happen to us all. It's really a very exciting future, provided we don't turn the planet into a nuclear fireball first."

PART THREE:
HEALING

THE REAL BIONIC MAN

By Dick Teresi

The rumor began in 1972. That's when Martin Caidin's SF novel *Cyborg* was published. The rumor intensified when ABC turned *Cyborg* into the popular television program *Six Million Dollar Man*. The hero of the tv series, Steve Austin, is an astronaut whose body was almost destroyed in a rocket-sled accident. But by using bits of plastic, titanium, sophisticated electronics, and a nuclear power pack, medical scientists put him back together again. Moreover, not only was old Steve restored to peak condition, he was given superhuman capabilities. He now leaps over buildings, hears conversations half a mile away, sees with zoom-lens accuracy, and resists physical assaults that would fell a water buffalo.

It all adds up to good fun on the tube.

But the rumor is this: Many people speculate—and it's even been reported in the press—that the basic story line of Steve Austin is true. That somewhere—perhaps in a supersecret Houston laboratory, or hidden among the serpentine medical facilities of the National Institutes of Health in Bethesda, Maryland—there exists a team of scientists who are churning out Cyborgs at an assembly-line rate.

In search of the real Six Million Dollar Man, I went to Salt Lake City, home of the University of Utah, which has the most comprehensive bioengineering program in America. Utah has in fact already outclassed the Six Million Dollar Man in at least one respect—cost. This year the university will spend $2.4 million more than was spent on the theoretical Steve Austin, a total of $8.4 million, on bioengineering, the application of space-age technology to the repair and maintenance of the human body. And Utah employs more than 360 engineers, medical scientists, and technicians who work directly on what are popularly called "bionics" projects.

I talked to Stephen C. Jacobsen, director of the university's Projects and Design Lab and inventor of many outrageously futuristic devices, including a "thinking" artificial arm. He had a simple response to the claim that the government has a secret Cyborg laboratory.

"Bullshit," said Jacobsen. "If the government already has a Cyborg, well then, they're wasting a lot of money on us." He refers to the fact that most of Utah's bioengineering budget comes from federal grants and contracts.

Members of the bioengineering team at Utah agree that the future lies not in building Cyborgian robots, but in developing prostheses that mimic human body parts as closely as possible. Their research is focused on understanding how the body works and how to duplicate its physiology.

The university entered the field 14 years ago and in 1967 hired one of the pioneers of bioengineering, Willem J. Kolff, to head its artificial organs division. The Dutch-born Dr. Kolff invented the first artificial kidney during World War II. Working under near-secret conditions in the Nazi-occupied Netherlands, he saved the lives of end-stage kidney patients who, before his invention, would have been doomed. Today at Utah his mission remains unchanged.

"Our aim," says Kolff, "is to restore people." And there are few places where a better job of it is being done. Utah boasts spectacular programs in artificial vision and hearing, the most successful artificial heart project in the world, a new polymer-implant center that's developing plastic-like blood vessels, bladders, testicles, and other organs, and a whole assortment of other bioengineering marvels aimed at improving medical care. But for you Cyborg fans, let's begin with the device that's the most suggestive of science fiction—the Utah arm.

"I'm not trying to be obnoxious," said Stephen Jacobsen as he clipped an electronic sensor to my forearm, "but this is the best artificial arm ever made." The electrode on my arm, explained Jacobsen, picks up electromyographic (EMG) signals. "Every time you flex a muscle, electrical activity is produced on the surface of your skin. It's crawling all over you."

A wire led from the sensor on my forearm to a one-kilogram (2.2 pound) artificial arm, which Jacobsen held just above the elbow by its stump socket. I held my arm straight at my side with my wrist relaxed. But when I flexed my wrist and raised my hand, the artificial arm also moved upward, bending at the elbow. When I dropped my hand, the Utah arm dropped. Crudely speaking the electrode had picked up the EMG signals on my forearm and transmitted them to a minicomputer in the arm, which in turn commanded the arm's electric motor to flex it up or down at the elbow.

Of course, the arm is meant to be used by an amputee, in which case it is fitted over the patient's stump. Electrodes would pick up the amputee's EMG signals from his limb remnant and from his shoulders, chest, and back on the affected side. Besides elbow flexion, the amputee can operate three other joint-movements: humeral rotation, wrist rotation, and hand closure.

The beauty of the Utah arm is that an armless person doesn't have to be taught how to use it. "The amputee has muscles left in his stump that don't pull on anything anymore. But they're still connected to his brain. We pick up those signals and have them control the arm," explains Jacobsen. "He doesn't have to do anything unnatural, like wink to close his hand." In effect, all the amputee must do is think and act as if he had a real arm and use his muscles as he did before amputation. The Utah arm does the rest.

Jacobsen believes in developing medical devices to the point where companies will want to pick them up and sell them to the public. And he often becomes so enthusiastic when ticking off the arm's commercial attributes that he sounds a bit like a high-class Cuisinart salesman:

"It has a nice, cosmetic exterior, a nice weight. It's quiet in operation, smooth, and doesn't pinch or cut clothing. It will go fast, slow, and lock in place. It will lift three pounds and support fifty pounds. It has a great electronic package. The batteries are easily replaceable by the amputee; even the circuits can be removed and replaced. It's repairable, maintainable, and can be sold at a reasonable price: *under* three thousand dollars."

Jacobsen's style, though, stems simply from his desire to get ideas from the lab out into society. "So many ideas," he says, "just stay locked up in universities. The public pays for the research but never receives the benefits. It's like pouring money down a hole."

The Utah arm will be ready for home use in less than a year, according to Jacobsen.

Right now it is still being tested in the Project and Design Lab. Several amputees have used the arm, but never outside the lab. Jacobsen and his staff fit a dozen or so electrodes to each subject. Then they use a computer to adjust the arm's movements to the amputee's EMG signals. Each arm must be electronically tailored to its wearer.

But recently, while working out equations for the arm's control system, Jacobsen made what he calls an "awe-inspiring" discovery. He noticed the possibility of making a feedback loop in the circuitry. What you'd then have is an adapter-controller in the arm that would automatically adapt its movements to the amputee. "You'd just slap an arm on somebody," says Jacobsen, "and they'd reach an agreement about how they were going to behave."

Even though the Utah arm may be the best artificial arm in the world, Jacobsen scoffs at the better-than-human, bionic concept of his work. Recently a major encyclopedia company made a film about the Project and Design Lab. Jacobsen is still reeling from the results. "Jesus, I just saw a copy of it and its the absolute worst," he says. "The narrator turned out to be the actor who stars in *The Bionic Woman* [the tv show] and he was standing the whole time in front of this stupid panel of flashing lights that was obviously out of some tv series because the discs in the computer didn't spin right." The effect of this kind of publicity is an illusion that amputees fitted with these new devices will be bionic supermen.

Those people expecting a Cyborg-strong arm have a long wait ahead of them. The Utah arm can lift little more than one kilogram (three pounds). And while Jacobsen says a one-kilogram lift is adequate for 95 percent of all normal human arm activity, it;s still a far cry from a real arm's capacity, somewhere between 23 and 45 kilograms (50-100 pounds).

To make the arm more competitive with its human counterpart, Jacobsen says four technological advances must be made. First, he needs better motors (compared to muscles, says Jacobsen, "motors are crummy"). Second, he needs a way to attach the prosthesis directly to the bone so it can support more weight. Other breakthroughs needed are a way to hook into the amputee's nerves for better control of the arm and some kind of feedback system so the wearer can tell without looking at it what his arm is doing.

But the Utah team understands the basic physiology of arm movement. And in this respect Jacobsen says the arm is designed as far as it can go. "We don't need a fancy new designer. We need new technology."

Michael G. Mladejovsky (mal-YOFF-ski) has

the opposite problem. Director of the Neuroprostheses Program at Utah, he's been working on developing an artificial vision system for almost a decade. He says facetiously that building a device that serves as an eye is a "mere technological problem." He could build it right now with existing electronic hardware and techniques . . . if only he knew what it was supposed to *do*.

There's the rub. No one quite yet knows what happens in the brain that allows people to see. But no one has come closer to finding out than the scientists at Utah.

William H. Dobelle started Utah's artificial vision program in 1969. Dobelle's role was to handle the physiological side — what goes on inside the visual cortex — while Mladejovsky handled the computer-hardware end of the project.

They had been inspired by a 1968 discovery in England that blind persons, as well as people who see, can perceive spots of light called phosphenes when the visual cortex at the back of the brain is stimulated with electricity. These phosphenes usually appear as bright, white dots — patients describe them as "starlight" — but sometimes they're yellow-green, red, or blue-white.

The Utah team's idea was this: if you could stimulate the cortex of a blind person in an orderly way, you could draw pictures in his mind composed of phosphenes. And, in a way, that's exactly what they've done — by using electronics and surgery.

Three years ago Dobelle and Mladejovsky found a willing subject, named Craig, who had been blinded in a gunshot accident. Craig agreed to some very scary brain surgery. The Utah team fashioned a two-inch square Teflon wafer studded with 64 electrodes. Surgeons separated hemispheres of Craig's brain to expose the visual area, placed the wafer against it, then let the two brain halves drop back into position, holding the wafer in place. A wire connected to the implant was threaded through a hole in the back of the skull, then snaked forward between the skull and scalp to a buttonlike connector that protruded (and still protrudes today) above Craig's right ear.

Mladejovsky was thus able to connect the electrodes implanted in Craig's brain to a computer, which in turn was connected to a tv camera. The camera was pointed at a simple image, such as a piece of masking tape on a dark-green screen. The visual image was simplified by the computer and carried as electrical impulses to Craig's brain.

It worked. He was able to see the strip of tape as a white line and tell whether it was vertical, horizontal, or tilted at a 45-degree angle. The Utah team also stimulated letters of the Braille alphabet in Craig's brain, and he was able to visually read simple sentences like, "He had a cat and a ball." Mladejovsky found there was no limit on speed; he could flash new letters to Craig faster than Craig could read by the normal tactile Braille method.

But blind people don't want artificial vision for reading but rather for mobility. They want to be able to navigate without being led around by another person or a dog. They want to find their way through unfamiliar territory without tripping over obstacles; they want to spot curbs, doors, follow crosswalks, see automobiles. Can this be done? Probably.

Mladejovsky foresees building a miniaturized television camera mounted in a dummy pair of glasses. The electronics needed to convert the images would be carried on a belt. A cable could be run from the electronics package up the person's back under his clothes and then concealed under his hair, finally connecting to the implant's exterior "button" and to the camera-carrying eyeglasses.

What would the blind person see? Mladejovsky believes phosphene-dot moving pictures could be created, similar to those you see on electronic scoreboards in baseball and football stadiums. Only the images would be much cruder. The device implanted in Craig's brain contains 64 electrodes, which produce 42 phosphenes (you don't get a 1:1 ratio). The next step is an implant with 256 electrodes.

Assuming that it will produce 256 useful phosphenes, which it might not, you'd still only be able to create crude, silhouettelike images. But they would be adequate for navigation. Mladejovsky showed me two pictures, each composed of only 256 dots. One I could make out clearly as a man's bearded face. The second image, a pair of scissors, I didn't recognize. But Mladejovsky emphasizes that the blind person would have other clues to guide him in recognizing objects — sound, smell, an object's size in proportion to its surroundings. If he was standing at a crosswalk and he saw a large oblong object getting closer and closer, accompanied by the sound of an internal combustion engine, he would know enough to get out of its way.

Mladejovsky thinks that eventually they may be able to stimulate as many as 500 useful phosphenes in a person's visual cortex. Of course, many problems have to be worked out first.

William Dobelle recently left Utah to head the artificial organs department of Columbia University in New York City, where he continues his work, trying to solve the physiological mysteries of eyesight. Craig is still part of the project, shuttling back and forth between Utah and New York.

"In the meantime," says Mladejovsky, "I'm just biding my time. I can't do anything more until Dobelle, or somebody like him, can finally sit down and set up concrete specifications for what the artificial vision device should do." When that day comes, Mladejovsky and his colleagues in Utah's Microcircuit Lab are prepared to build the 'Utah eyes.' "A mere technological problem," Mladejovsky repeats.

The artificial hearing project at Utah is quite similar to the eyesight project. Electrodes have been implanted in the cochlear membranes of the inner ears of four deaf volunteers.

Mladejovsky and other Utah researchers are stimulating the cochlea with electrical signals to create sounds of varying pitch and loudness. As with artificial vision, the ultimate goal is to understand how human hearing works, and then build miniaturized computer circuitry that can be used in a portable hearing device. (The computer used in the artificial hearing experiments, like that used for artificial vision, is presently gigantic — 2.7 meters by 2.7 meters high.)

While artificial hearing may not sound as spectacular as artificial vision, Mladejovsky claims it is a much more difficult venture because deaf subjects have great trouble communicating what they're experiencing. It is difficult to describe subtle variations in pitch and loudness, and most subjects are mute and must communicate by writing or sign language.

The team's biggest break came when they found a willing subject who was deaf in one ear only. Paul, the unilaterally deaf subject, has electrodes implanted in his deaf ear. When his cochlea is stimulated electronically, he tunes an audio oscillator to produce a matching sound on his good ear. This way he can tell the researchers exactly what they're producing with their electrical signals.

But Mladejovsky admits that producing artificial hearing is much more difficult than anyone had suspected.

Donald Olsen, a veterinarian in Utah's artificial heart lab, gently kicked a sleepy looking calf named Theodore. It was enough to bring Theodore rapidly to his feet. "See," said Olsen, "this calf is perfectly healthy." Theodore did, in fact, look very healthy. The only thing distinguishing him from a normal calf was an array of air hoses sticking out of his side. The hoses connected Theodore to an external compressed-air pump that powered his artificial heart. Some 85 days earlier, Olsen had removed the calf's real heart and replaced it with a molded polyurethane model called the Jarvik-7. Designed by Robert Jarvik, head of Utah's heart program, Jarvik-7 is similar to Jarvik-5, the plastic heart that holds the world longevity record for artificial hearts. It kept a Holstein calf named Abebe alive in the Utah facilities for over six months; 184 days to be exact. Abebe died in May 1977, not because of a malfunction, but simply because he was a growing young cow and had outgrown the heart. (Calves are used because their cardiac output is similar to man's, they are good animals to operate on and they are far cheaper — at $200 apiece — than gorillas or baboons.)

Theodore's Jarvik-7 brings Utah one step closer to artificial heart implantation in man because, unlike Jarvik-5, it is the exact size needed for a human being.

An artificial heart has been implanted in man on only one occasion. That was Dr. Denton Cooley's controversial operation on Haskell Karp on 1969. Karp survived only a span of hours with the implant.

Since then, blood pumps have been used as temporary-assist devices to keep cardiac patients alive for short periods of time, but there have been no more total replacements.

This hiatus is partly due to now stricter federal regulations for all medical devices to be used in human beings, as well as obviously due in part to technical problems still to be worked out. Perhaps most important, however, is the recent decision by the National Advisory Heart Council to give left-ventricular-assist devices (LVADs) first priority and to deemphasize total hearts. This has brought a partial drying-up of funds for the Utah heart team.

Willem Kolff differs strongly with the Council's philosophy. If the patient is sick enough to need an LVAD, claims Kolff, he really needs a whole new pump. Kolff feels that an assist pump cannot sustain a heart patient whose condition is so bad that all conventional remedies have failed.

The drying-up of funds has temporarily killed one of Donald Olsen's favorite projects, the nuclear heart. Olsen favors hearts with a built-in power source because they offer the patient independence. He also feels there's less chance of infection because you don't have to run electric wires or air hoses into the body.

An electric heart will probaably be the next step but, Olsen says, the batteries would have to be recharged every three to four hours. A nuclear-powered heart, on the other hand, could run 40 years on a small supply of plutonium 238.

There is one potential problem, however. While plutonium 238, unlike plutonium 239, is not fissionable (you can't make a bomb out of it), it *is* highly carcinogenic and could be used to poison a city's water supply. The nuclear heart conjures up a horror scenario of terrorists kidnapping several cardiac patients and killing them for their plutonium capsules.

Kolff is not overly enthusiastic about the nuclear heart. He doesn't share Olsen's pessimism over running wires into the human body and calls the electric heart a perfectly sane solution. The power pack would be worn outside the body, with wires leading inside. When asked about the risk of infection, Kolff said, "So what? We're talking about patients with a life expectancy of five minutes." Kolff also made note of Dobelle's success in implanting wires into Craig's head and leaving them for three years with no sign of infection.

Another solution would be to induce electric current through the skin. Two coils—one inside the body, one outside—would transmit power from an external battery to the heart's motor.

The heart isn't the only internal organ that can fail in the human body. Blood vessels, nerves, bile ducts, ureters, bladders, and lungs also fall victim to disease and injury. Utah's plan: repair and replace these damaged tissues with synthetic plastics and rubber. Armed with a $1.4 million federal grant, the university recently set up the nation's first Biomedical Engineering Center for Polymer Implants.

Donald J. Lyman, director of the new center, has already implanted in dogs tiny blood vessel grafts made of a new polyurethanelike material. Very large grafts made of Dacron have been used for years to repair major blood vessels such as the human aorta. But Dacron and similar materials are too rigid and fail quickly when used for smaller arteries and veins.

What's needed is a flexible material that has enough give as the blood pulsates through it. That's exactly what Lyman and his staff of 20 have created. The flexible grafts in dogs are only three millimeters in diameter—smaller than needed for humans—and have lasted 18 months. Polymer implants in humans are expected within a year.

Lyman explains that 80 percent of the human body is made of polymers, which are simply very large molecules (Europeans call them macromolecules). DNA, for example, is a polymer. And Lyman's office reminds one of something out of Watson and Crick and the search for *The Double*

Helix. The day I visited him, it was cluttered with atomic models that looked like long chains of different-colored plastic baseballs. One 1 2/3-meter-long model had claimed sole possession of the office couch. Lyman said it represented only 1/20th of a polymer he was "designing."

That's basically what the center is doing: "We're mapping implants atom by atom." Lyman and his colleagues are creating brand-new synthetic polymers, which he said could be loosely described as plastics or rubberlike, in order to find the perfect implant materials. Lyman expects his polymers to have mind-boggling characteristics. First, they must survive far longer in the human body than conventional implant materials. Second, they must eventually degenerate. Initially, this seems contradictory.

But Lyman's plan makes infinite sense. Polymer blood vessels, ureters, bladders, or whatever must last long enough for the patient to survive. However, Lyman believes only a few synthetics can last forever in the body. Human tissue is constantly changing while the implant is not. The trick then is to create materials that will encourage tissue growth on their outside surfaces. In this way, a blood vessel could be implanted, and over a number of years, it would slowly degrade while natural polymers would take its place, eventually replacing it entirely. In other words, you could rebuild a man's insides with Utah implants and in, say, ten years you could cut him open and find nothing synthetic — only normal, natural tissue. The real goal of implantation, then, is regeneration.

Once the right polymers are invented, Lyman

foresees building any number of body parts: lungs, an esophagus and trachea, skin, testicles, fallopian tubes, even nerves. "Blood vessels are rather simple," says Lyman. "They're really just pipes. The bladder is a bag. But nerves are more like telephone wires." Even so, Lyman plans to make, implant, and regenerate nerves. Eventually.

It seems odd that with all the medical-science heavyweights concentrated in the establishment East and on the innovative West Coast that the most sophisticated bioengineering effort in the U. S. is going on in Salt Lake City. At first I suspected a religious motive, considering the overwhelming influence of the Church of Latter-Day Saints on the city. That idea was quickly dispelled.

"Salt Lake is a beautiful city for skiers and backpackers," said one researcher who asked not to be identified. "With all these beautiful mountains, you can put up with almost any number of Mormons."

Dr. Kolff gives a more mundane reason for Utah's success: money. The university has set up Kolff in a special position that allows him great freedom in acquiring federal funds. Kolff reports directly to the vice-president in charge of research.

The univeristy's bioengineering program is not without its fund-raising problems, however. The school is sometimes out-maneuvered by more powerful and better-connected rivals in the fight for federal money. I mentioned Michael E. DeBakey, perhaps the most famous name in heart research, to Dr. Kolff and obviously hit a sore spot. President Nixon awarded DeBakey's team at Baylor College of Medicine in Houston a real plum several years ago: the opportunity to work with Soviet scientists on a joint U. S.-U. S. S. R. artificial heart project. Kolff claims Baylor only got the job because of DeBakey's tremendous power in Washington. "They sent the least successful heart group in the country to Moscow," said Kolff. While that may ring of sour grapes, DeBakey's longevity results with artificial hearts *are* rather meager when compared to those of Utah's heart program.

And there's another funding problem. Kolff says Utah sometimes suffers from the government's peer-review system of awarding grants. "We're so far ahead in our field," says Kolff immodestly, "that it's sometimes hard to find peers."

And that pretty much describes the bioengineering effort at Utah — peerless. The Six Million Dollar Man as portrayed on television will probably never exist. But the $8.4 Million Man is alive and well and living in Salt Lake City.

OTHER MARVELOUS MEDICAL MIRACLES AT UTAH

THE INSTANT BLOOD TEST

Utah scientists are on the verge of eliminating one of the biggest annoyances of a visit to the doctor — the blood test that requires a wait of several hours to a week before you get the results. Often, a doctor must send your blood off to lab, and you must make a second appointment — and pay a second fee—before you can be properly diagnosed and treated.

Bioengineers Stanley D. Moss and Jiri Janata think the Chemfet, or Superprobe, will end all that. About the size of a needle point, it's a microprocessor chip (like those used in pocket calculators) to which a tiny chemical membrane of the type used in medical labs for blood tests has been bonded. What you have then is a tiny computer that instantaneously measures concentrations of vital blood chemicals.

Let's say the doctor wants to know how much potassium you have in your bloodstream. He would take a syringe fitted with a Chemfet and stick it in your arm. But he would draw no blood. A desk top computer connected to the syringe would display an immediate readout of the blood's potassium level.

The Utah scientists have already built a prototype that measures potassium and are close to making pH and calcium probes. Next on the horizon will be fluoride and oxygen Chemfets. Moss says that a different Chemfet will not be be needed for each chemical measurement. He's confident they can fit at least six, and possibly ten, different membranes on one computer chip.

Chemfets have already been used in testing rhesus monkeys, dogs, and cats. Moss believes it will be a few years yet before they have an FDA-approved device.

PAINLESS ANESTHESIA

One of the problems of painkillers is that it hurts like hell to get them when a needle is used. But the Dermatron, developed by Stephen Jacobsen and the Projects and Design Lab, delivers anesthesia without puncturing the skin. A band containing two electrodes and a dose of an anesthethic drug is strapped over the skin to be anesthetized. The band is connected by cable to a power unit the size of a pocket calculator. By a process called iontophoresis, the drug is driven through the skin into the tissue. It's painless and avoids possible infection and irritation from standard needles.

The Dermatron has been used to anesthetize dialysis patients and those undergoing wart removal, minor finger surgery, and the draining of abscesses.

THE WEARABLE KIDNEY

When a person's kidneys fail, he must be hooked up to an artificial kidney, or dialysis machine, in order to cleanse his blood of urea and other toxic substances. The standard artificial kidney is about the size of a washing machine, and the patient must go to a hospital three or four times a week and sit for several hours while the apparatus filters waste from his blood.

Now Utah researchers have built an artificial kidney that can be worn right on the body. It weighs eight pounds and can be strapped down next to him. In either case, it allows the kidney patient infinitely more freedom and mobility than standard dialysis does. Even though the wearable kidney must be connected intermittently to an 18-liter tank, it still means dialysis patients can travel and lead more normal lives.

3-D TELEVISION FOR YOUR BODY

Utah scientists have built a "television" that transforms x-rays into three-dimensional images. Brent S. Baxter and Steven A. Johnson of the Advanced Imaging Methods Laboratory have already projected a realistic 3-D illusion of a human brain onto a television screen. It doesn't require special glasses as the old 3-D movies did, and several people can look at the image at the same time. The image also has parallax; that is, when you shift your head, you can see around the outside of the image, or you can bend down and look up into the image (or vice versa) and get a different view.

Baxter says the device could be used for air traffic control (creating 3-D pictures of planes over an airport), architectural design, and for making 3-D geological maps of potential ore beds. — *D.T.*

CELL DEFENDER

By Mike Edelhart

Joan Karafotas is one of the chosen few. This Illinois housewife is one of eight cancer victims to receive the world's first batches of genetically engineered interferon. Her treatment will help scientists determine whether interferon made from recombined DNA is safe enough for use in broader human experiments.

Karafotas's experience is the latest chapter in the continuing story of interferon, a substance that languished on the back shelves of science for more than two decades, but that has now been thrust to the forefront in the battle against cancer. Interferon has become a new media buzz word, its use now commonly linked to the treatment of the rich and the famous. When John Wayne was fading into his last sunset, what miracle drug did doctors consider to treat his cancer? Interferon. In the shah of Iran's final days what substance stood at the center of veiled transactions between Europe and Egypt? Interferon. Rumors like these have helped inflame speculation about the drug, scarcely diminished by the fact that both famed would-be recipients died.

But Joan Karafotas's treatment may have more substance and should shed more light on what role interferon will play in all our lives.

Interferon has followed a roller-coaster course to its present promising status, in which it is regarded as a potential magic bullet for cancer and as a treatment for a host of other serious diseases, including the common cold and rabies. In the beginning it was lionized as the new penicillin for viral infections. It then fell to near scientific anonymity, but now it has been dusted off and given a second chance for scientific prominence. What we will try to present here is a sober evaluation of its potential in therapy.

Interferon is a virus-fighting agent of unmatched range but problematical power. It has shown itself potent against every virus that nature or man has thrown against it. But it has also displayed limitations that keep it from becoming the wide-ranging preventive once hoped for.

As an antitumor drug, interferon displays exciting abilities against an ever-expanding array of tumors. It has caused complete remission in some tumors, such as non-malignant papilloma, and has caused cancerous tumors of at least a half-dozen varieties to shrink. The scarcity of the drug, however, has kept tests so small and brief that the conclusions drawn from them must be tentative at best. Interferon's apparent abilities to combat tumors are not conclusive, but the tests performed so far are highly suggestive. They indicate a substance that doesn't so much kill cancer as control it. And it is this notion, that a natural substance from our own bodies can somehow modify the behavior of raging cancer cells, that so excites researchers.

It is unlikely that interferon will prove to be the long-sought miracle drug against cancer. Instead, it will probably be a new weapon to be added to medicine's existing arsenal. "Interferon and other biological response modifiers will not replace traditional therapies, but they will enhance them," says Jordan Gutterman, who runs the interferon test program at Houston's M. D. Anderson Cancer Center.

A clear, comprehensive view of expectations for interferon comes from Mathilde Krim, a dynamo behind interferon's current push to the fore in research. At her tiny desk on the eleventh floor of Memorial Sloan-Kettering Cancer Center's main lab building on Manhattan's Upper East Side. Krim earnestly expounds on her favorite subject: "I don't claim that interferon will be the magic bullet for cancer. I don't know that there is such a thing, to tell you the truth. But what other substance, at so early a stage in its development, has shown so much promising activity against different—often highly resistant—strains of cancer? And can anyone name another cancer therapy that has shown so few side effects—all of them apparently reversible?"

Krim accepts the fact that many scientists, even some working in the field, have serious doubts about interferon's effectiveness. "What we have to determine is the level of activity," she says. "We have to improve our knowledge of the dose, the length of treatment. And it's important that we improve the purity of the material we're working with.

"Remember," she adds, "the first patients treated with penicillin died. The situations are similar. There may be different opinions, but mine is that interferon will rank at least as high as chemotherapy and radiation as a cancer treatment. And the beauty is that it can be added to the others and provide benefits they can't."

Interferon is a protein our bodies produce regularly. It protects our cells from the ravages of invasion. When cells are threatened by a virus, they turn into interferon factories in order to save as many surrounding cells as possible. Interferon is the body's first line of defense against a concentrated assault. It can't hold off attackers forever, but it fends them off while greater forces muster for the counterattack.

The spread of malignant cells seems to be linked somehow to a suppression of the body's normal ability to fight off unnatural elements. Dr. Norman Finter, of Britain's Burroughs-Wellcome Laboratory, believes that cancers manage to sneak past the interferon control system. "It's an insidious change in the natural cell the body doesn't recognize. The change from a normal cell to a cancer cell is a slight mutation," he says. "Then there's another mutation and another, and then the body picks it up because it has become sufficiently different, but it's already too late to control without outside help. The mutation has escaped the system that stimulates production of interferon until the cancer establishes itself."

When this happens, the answer is to use laboratory-produced interferon to trigger an immune response. Interferon injections can produce significant antitumor effects in mice, apparently by heightening the body's own natural defenses against such cells. In culture dishes, however, the protein has little or no effect against cancer. The secret? Interferon does not engage in hand-to-hand combat with malignant cells. It leaves the dirty work to a strange bodily enforcer called the NK (for Natural Killer) cells. How they work is not yet understood, but what they do is pretty clear.

NK cells float through the body on constant alert against abnormal cells. Like a SWAT team, they rush in with high firepower when the situation is on the verge of getting out of hand. The presence of interferon in the vicinity of a tumor is believed to act like a beacon on a foggy night. Patrolling NK cells pick up the distress signal and move toward the area. Meanwhile the interferon slows cell division to hold down the growth of the invader until help arrives. The NK cells eradicate the tumor itself, though how they do this remains hazy.

The NK-interferon partnership strikes down viruses in a similar manner. When the body recognizes virus-infected cells as alien, interferon floods the area and calls in NK cells for a massive mop-up.

For all its potency, interferon has little staying

power in the body. From an early peak, interferon fades steadily away and is gone entirely the day after it was induced. On the one hand, this worries researchers because it raises the possibility that long-term treatment with interferon might generate dangerous side effects. The body may be protecting itself from these developments by wiping interferon out of the system quickly. Under some circumstances, though, the fading interferon pattern has been found to help treatment. If some cells are given a small dose of interferon and then challenged with a second larger dose after the first has begun to fade, the cells put out a startling spurt of interferon by themselves. This is called superinduction; its value is that it can extend limited interferon supplies by letting the body make up some of the virus-fighting supply itself.

If interferon can modulate the growth of tumors, why doesn't it nip cancer in the bud? It probably does, says Dr. Derek Burke, of Warwick University, in England. "You can easily say that interferon does work against cancer colonies in the body and we see only the cases where it fails. We know that you need multiple events in order to initiate a tumor. Each of the events is intrinsically rather unlikely. This is why cancer takes so long to develop, why cancer tends to be a disease of old age. All of this suggests that there is a mechanism for blocking these rather rare events and that the mechanism becomes less efficient as we become older.

"So maybe interferon is working and what we see in tumor growth is the breakdown in some rather subtle link in the immune system that is normally modulated by interferon."

Beyond cancer, the natural chemical has shown hints of startling activity in other areas of medicine. Immune responses that plague transplant recipients seem to be suppressed by properly applied interferon. At the same time interferon can increase immune protection for patients in danger of massive infection. Few medicines have demonstrated such remarkable flexibility. Preliminary lab studies in animals may even lead to interferon treatments for obesity and Down's syndrome. Plants make their own version of the protein to protect themselves, and some people's failure to produce interferon when under attack by certain low-level viruses might hold the key to understanding many chronic conditions.

Interferon is still proving itself in the scientific boondocks, but the clout of genetic engineering will soon pave the way for broad clinical tests. Until the hard-core data roll in, no one can be certain just how much of interferon's prowess is ingrained, how much is hopeful thinking, and how much is hype.

To put interferon into proper perspective, look back to the original wonder drug, penicillin. In the war-torn years of the early 1940s there were tremendous doubts about penicillin's commercial value. Despite its enormous potential, it was prohibitively costly to manufacture. Even with massive government support, pharmaceutical companies were reluctant to take the risks involved in developing new, improved methods of production. If it had not been for the needs of troops wounded in combat, penicillin might also have followed a 25-year course to prominence.

The doubt and trouble that afflicted penicillin a generation ago have given way to overwhelming praise and acceptance. Moreover, penicillin led to the creation of a whole new family of medicines, many of which far outstrip their progenitor in power and range of effectiveness.

In all these respects the future of interferon will likely be much the same. In their later years, today's young adults will almost certainly find interferon among the common treatments prescribed by physicians. Some of these future patients will be given the opportunity to try new "biologicals," sophisticated hormonelike proteins being tested to supplant interferon as the sole cell-modulating medication.

When these same people years hence feel colds coming on, they will get prescriptions for interferon nasal spray. It will be kept under prescription to protect those prone to allergic reactions.

When they are stricken by chronic or unusually severe virus infections, interferon will be used to hold the disease in check until a vaccine can be prepared or until the patient is better able to fight it off. In a few cases interferon therapy strong enough to wipe out the infection will be used. Most often doctors will want to give the patient time to develop antibodies to the disease, so that it won't recur.

After organ transplantation, interferon will serve as a lifeline that wards off virus infections and inhibits the body's natural tendency to reject the foreign tissue. Treatment may be required for days, weeks, or even a lifetime. The side effects won't matter much. lWhatever they are, they will be preferable to the alternative: tissue rejection, followed by death.

The treatment for cancer will be more akin to today's approach to diabetes or several prostate problems. Cancer won't ever be pleasant — not by any stretch of the imagination. It will still be traumatic and dangerous, but the medication will offer effective therapy without deadly or permanent side effects.

A patient might still be sent into surgery or radiation for the treatment of the initial tumor. Then interferon therapy will begin. The protein will help prevent metastasis — the dreaded spread of cancer to other parts of the body. It will also keep the patient strong and free of virus infections, so that other treatments will have less sting. By boosting the body's natural immune system during this critical phase, interferon promises dramatically to reduce the death toll of cancer.

Krim notes that "the trouble with today's treatment is that we can do very little about getting rid of residual cancer cells once the primary tumor has been attacked. Because of their enormous side effects we hesitate to use chemotherapy or radiation when definite signs of cancer aren't present. A recurrence can get a toehold before we go in and try to stop it. In the future, I think, we should follow surgery with interferon to strengthen the patient's defenses so he can get rid of his residual cancer cells before they can form colonies. I believe it will significantly decrease the percentage of recurrence."

When will interferon emerge from the labs and clinics and be placed on doctors' shelves? Not fast enough to make very many people happy. The development of new drugs takes time because no one — not in science, medicine, government, or business — wants to let a mistake jeopardize the lives of millions of trusting patients.

Today researchers can say without hesitation that interferon works to some extent. What they must be able to say before they can bring a drug to the market is: Interferon works here and doesn't work there. Interferon performs better here than it does there. Interferon given this way is more effective than interferon given that way. Interferon should never be given to this kind of person, but it can always be safely given to that kind of person.

And, most important, scientists need to know that interferon works this way for specific, identifiable reasons.

The protein must be studied and understood before it can be unleashed in the maze of situations that confront doctors in practive. This process takes years, and it can be altered by the unexpected in the long stretch ahead. Given smooth sailing, however, interferon's course should follow a timetable like this:

1981: Genetically engineered interferon is produced, examined by government agencies, and approved for limited human testing. More detailed reports of clinical trials with natural interferon will appear.

1982: Results of genetically engineered interferon studies will begin to trickle out. The aggressive companies behind these tests will push for government approval to market it as quickly as possible. If the findings look good, the companies will get it. Interferon will flood the commercial arena, and its price will plummet.

1983: Drawing upon the huge supply of interferon, companies begin testing, and shortly thereafter marketing, interferon nasal sprays for restricted use. Interferon becomes accepted as a treatment against rabies, eliminating the painful series of injections now used to prevent the disease's deadly onset.

1984: With interferon's properties now well delineated, genetic-engineering companies will undertake the development of second-generation biological drugs. Some are more specific in action than interferon, some broader and milder. Some act only in certain parts of the body.

1985: An aging scientist, in his memoirs, will look back and write: "Amazing as it may seen today, in the late 1970s and early 1980s there were many people, even many scientists, who doubted that interferon would ever have a role in medicine. If only they could be here now."

AN END TO PAIN

By Jonathan B. Tucker

A brutal car accident left Barbara Loew with excruciating pain in her neck and back. At first her doctor thought it was severe whiplash. Months passed, but the pain never lessened. She tried sleeping tablets, Valium, hundreds of painkillers. None could relieve the agony that had become a daily part of her existence. Like 20 million other American victims of chronic pain, Barbara undertook a frustrating search for relief.

Several years after the accident, her doctor told her of a revolutionary new drug. "I haven't prescribed it to any of my other patients yet," he said hesitantly, "but the drug appears to be totally safe—it's nonaddictive, there's no buildup of tolerance, and it doesn't put you to sleep. Furthermore, you become desensitized only to the pain that bothers you. For instance, you'd still feel a burn if you placed your hand on a hot stove. Since your back pains have been unresponsive to any other medications, why not give it a try?"

To Barbara's astonishment, there were only two pills in the glass container given her by the pharmacist — a perscription that was supposed to last a month. The directions read, "Take one tablet every 24 hours." By the end of the second day, she was discouraged — nothing had happened. But on the morning of the third day, the aching pain that had plagued her for so long was gone. Even more startling, the relief lasted for a whole month.

"How does it work?" Barbara asked her doctor.

"It's really your body that does the work," he explained. "The body has its own defense against pain — an opiatelike substance naturally produced in the brain that controls the amount of pain you feel. The drug I gave you gradually increased the levels of this brain chemical to provide long-lasting relief."

Although Barbara Loew's story is fictitious, preliminary tests conducted on a group of chronic-pain patients last year indicate that the wonder drug in this story may already exist. The potent analgesic properties of this drug were not discovered accidentally. Rather, the finding was precipitated by rapid developments in our understanding of pain only during the last decade — advances that promise to provide powerful new tools for treating chronic pain by exploiting the body's own pain-inhibitory system. But before we can discuss these exciting developments, we first need to know more about pain itself.

Pain physiologists have long debated whether specific pain sensors exist or whether pain results from the excessive stimulation of sensory cells that respond to touch, temperature, and pressure. This question was only recently resolved when physiology professor Edward R. Perl of the University of North Carolina School of Medicine identified nerve endings that are activated only if the stimulus is of sufficient intensity to be painful. These nerve endings have fine interwoven branches and are located in the deep layers of the skin, the internal organs, the membrane covering the bones, the cornea of the eyes, and the pulp of the teeth.

When a region of the skin is injured, the death of the cells in that area is believed to cause the liberation of chemicals associated with inflammation, such as histamine and bradykinin; these substances in turn trigger volleys of nerve impulses in the pain sensors. One of the actions of aspirin is to inhibit the manufacture of bradykinin, so that the generation of pain is blocked at the wound site.

The impulses generated in the pain fibers enter the spinal cord and travel through it to the cerebral cortex, where the location of the painful stimulus is pinpointed on the body surface. The limbic system — a doughnut-shaped region surrounding the core of the brain — appears to mediate the emotional component of pain. The prefrontal cortex located just behind the forehead may also participate in this aspect of the pain experience. Frontal lobotomy, a type of psychosurgery formerly used to treat chronic pain, involved severing the connections between the prefrontal cortex and the rest of the brain. After the operation patients reported that the pain was still there but that it didn't bother them; they simply no longer cared about it and often forgot that it was there. But the personality changes resulting from lobotomy — loss of spontaneity, reduced intelligence, and lowered responsiveness — often made the cure more terrible than the disease.

Surprisingly, the brain itself is totally insensitive to pain. Although it interprets pain signals from the rest of the body, the brain can be cut or burned without any conscious sensation, and most brain operations are performed with the patient fully awake. Headaches do not orginate in the brain itself but rather from a tightening of the muscles of the scalp owing to nervous tension or, in the case of migraine, from the pressure of swollen blood vessels within the skull against the sensitive membrane that sheathes the brain.

A major breakthrough in the understanding of the physiology of pain came in 1973 with the discovery in the central nervous system of specific receptors, or attachment sites, for morphine and other drugs of the opiate family. These "opiate receptors" were highly concentrated in regions of the brain and spinal cord traditionally associated with the perception of pain, such as the central gray matter of the brain stem and the limbic system.

As it typically happens in science, the answer to one puzzling question — how an age-old drug exerts its influence — soon presented a more baffling mystery. Why did the brains of human beings and other mammals evolve with receptors for a chemical in the sap of the opium poppy? A rapid series of discoveries soon revealed that the brain manufactures its own opiates. The unparalleled painkilling properties of morphine (the active ingredient of opium) are made possible because the drug mimics the natural opiates produced in the brain. As Stanford University pharmacologist Avram Goldstein points out, it is "one of nature's most bizarre coincidences" that the configuration of a natural chemical in the brain should match that of a substance found in the opium poppy.

The first of the brain's opiates to be discovered was termed enkephalin (from the Greek, meaning "in the head") and consists of a chain of five amino acids — the building blocks of protein. Although enkephalin chains are destroyed very rapidly by enzymes in the brain, chemical analogues of enkephalin have been prepared in the laboratory that are resistant to enzymatic breakdown. These analogues stimulate pain suppression when injected into the brain or the bloodstream of experimental animals. They are about three times as potent as morphine.

Another potent morphinelike substance, dubbed beta-endorphin ("the morphine within"), has been found in the pituitary gland at the base of the brain. Beta-endorphin appears to be a hormone that is released directly into the bloodstream, which carries it to specific target organs. Because beta-endorphin is released at the same time as the "stress hormone" ACTH, it is thought to play an important role in the body's defensive reactions to physical trauma and stress.

Pharmacology professor Solomon H. Snyder and his colleagues at the Johns Hopkins University School of Medicine recently investigated yet another brain chemical with pain killing properties. Called neurotensin, it is a chain of 13 amino acids. Like enkephalin, neurotensin is localized in brain regions that integrate information about pain and emotion. Although its precise function in modulating pain has yet to be determined, a recent study by the Merck pharmaceuticals company has shown neurotensin to be 1000 times more potent than enkephalin in relieving pain.

The discovery of natural opiate substances in the brain has provided new clues to how some very old pain remedies —from acupuncture to witch doctor's craft—may actually work. If the wisdom of the ancient Chinese was ever in doubt, certainly their methods of exploiting the brain's natural opiates in the treatment of pain and suffering were highly advanced. The first method the Chinese introduced was, of course, the smoking of opium, which no doubt became popular initially more for its euphoric properties than as a pain killer. The other method—acupuncture— has long aroused the suspicions of Western skeptics. Now, 2300 years after the ancient art was first developed, a link has been found between its anesthetic action and the opiates the brain produces.

David Mayer of the Medical College of Virginia subjected normal people to experimental pain caused by electrical stimulation of their teeth and found that acupuncture effectively raised the pain threshold. He then gave the subjects naloxone (a drug that blocks the action of enkephalin) and found that it significantly reduced the analgesic effects of acupuncture. This finding suggests that the stimulation of nerve endings by acupuncture needles triggers the release of enkephalin in the brain or spinal cord, thereby raising the pain threshold.

Nonetheless, faith in acupuncture may be an additional factor in its success. It has long been known that a patient's expectations may affect his response to treatment. The success of the witch doctor, often the most highly esteemed member of primitive tribes, may be largely attributable to the patient's belief in the cure. Modern researchers call this phenomenon the "placebo effect." Nearly one third of all patients recuperating from severe postsurgical pain report marked relief after being given a placebo — an inert compound such as a sugar pill or saline solution that the patient genuinely believes is a potent analgesic. ("Placebo comes from the Latin "I shall please.")

Evidence now suggests that the placebo effect is not just in the mind but also in the physical brain. Again, the natural opiates produced by the brain seem to be involved. Researchers at the University of California at San Francisco gave placebos to patients who suffered pain after wisdom-tooth extractions. As expected, the placebo brought about a significant reduction of pain in about one third of the patients. When these patients were subsequently given a drug that inhibits the actions of beta-endorphin, their pain increased back to almost the same level reported by patients who had not responded to the placebo in the first place.

Why placebos trigger the brain to release internal opiates in some patients but not in others remains a mystery. Researchers following this line of investigation speculate that stress may be the crucial factor. Indeed, two related observations — that patients under extreme stress often respond best to placebos, and that beta-endorphin is released from the pituitary simultaneously with the stress hormone ACTH — certainly lend plausibility to this theory. The role of beta-endorphin in stress may also explain peculiar aspects of pain tolerance, such as how athletes in the midst of competition and soldiers in battle can sustain severe injuries without becoming aware until later that they have been hurt. "One feels a single cut from a surgeon's scalpel," wrote Montaigne in the seventeenth century, "more than ten strokes of the sword in the heat of battle."

Could individuals learn to consciously control the release of opiates within their own bodies? Followers of Eastern religions who practice self-discipline and meditation in order to achieve inner awareness have long known how to control involuntary responses such as heart rate, respiration, and body temperature. It would not be surprising to discover that the trancelike state Oriental mystics enter before walking over beds of burning hot coals or passing needles through their flesh somehow enables them to regulate the release of internal opiates. For less mystically oriented Westerners, biofeedback training may someday provide the key to gaining control over this seemingly involuntary response.

Man from the beginning has sought to conquer pain. Prehistoric skulls found in Britain, France, and Peru possess gaping holes drilled by Stone Age surgeons in an effort to purge the evil spirits held responsible for headache, and Egyptian mummies over 4000 years old show evidence of painful kidney abscesses and tooth decay. Our word *pain* comes from the Latin *poena*, meaning punishment, for the ancients believed that pain was a penalty inflicted by the gods on any mortal who incurred their wrath.

Despite a more rational basis for treatment today, the quest for pain relief still remains a major endeavor. In the U.S. alone, $10 billion is spent on analgesic drugs and surgical procedures each year.

Until recently, the only effective treatment of chronic pain involved cutting pain pathways in the brain or spinal cord, or severing the peripheral nerves where they enter the cord. But the cost for such relief was terribly high: a useless, endangered limb or, in the case of psychosurgery, reduced intelligence and adverse personality changes.

In the last decade, however, approaches to pain therapy have changed radically owing to our new knowledge of the body's own pain-suppressing system. There has been a move away from the surgical treatment of pain to the electrical stimulation of peripheral nerves and parts of the brain involved in the pain-inhibitory system. This is not altogether a new method: In the first century A.D., the Roman physician Scribonium Largus relieved the pain of headache and gout by applying a live electric fish to the aching spot until the part became numb.

Today, current is applied with electrodes taped to the skin or implanted directly in the spinal cord or the brain so that the patient can intermittently activate them when the pain becomes too severe. Although the technique has proved effective in relieving chronic pain unresponsive to other therapies, it is not known whether excessive stimulation will lead to a reduction in the analgesic response over time or whether the presence of permanent metal electrodes in the brain tissue will have adverse long-term effects.

A second development in the treatment of chronic pain has been to devise new drugs possessing the beneficial qualities of morphine without the bad ones. In 1680, the English physician Thomas Sydenham wrote: "Among the remedies which it has pleased Almighty God to give men to relieve his sufferings, none is so universal and efficacious as opium." Even today, in spite of all the thousands of painkillers available, the opiates remain the only class of analgesic drug powerful enough to treat severe pain.

Unfortunately, the toxicity and addictiveness of opium and its derivatives have greatly tempered much of the medical community's initial enthusiasm toward this class of drugs. The isolation of morphine from dried-opium powder in 1803 was followed shortly by the invention of the hypodermic syringe, greatly facilitating the administration of pure morphine to large numbers of wounded soldiers during the Civil War. This made opiate addiction a significant social problem in the U. S., and as is well known, the situation has now reached epidemic proportions.

Over the years, the continuing search for a nonaddicting synthetic opiate has been frustrated time and time again. In the 1890s, a German pharmaceuticals house introduced heroin, a semisynthetic form of morphine, as a nonaddicting opiate. It soon proved to be more addictive than the drug it was designed to replace, probably because it enters the brain more rapidly from the bloodstream. Similarly, in the 1940s Demerol became the most popular opiate analgesic in America, because it was thought to be nonaddicting. The growing number of Demerol addicts soon convinced the Bureau of Narcotics otherwise.

The recent discovery of the brain's own opiates naturally raised hopes that modified forms of these chemicals might provide the long-sought nonaddicting analgesics. Enkephalin was chosen for the preparation of analogues because it is only five amino acids long. But to produce a medically useful enkephalin, it first had to be stabilized so that it would not be immediately destroyed, and chemically modified so that it would pass through the "blood-brain barrier" into the brain. Chemists at the Sandoz drug company in Basel, Switzerland, overcame these formidable obstacles: They managed to stabilize the molecule and enhance its activity so that one enkephalin analogue, designated FK-33824, is 30,000 times more potent than enkephalin."

Excitement about enkephalin analogues was quickly dampened when it was found that they, too, are addictive. When rats are regularly treated with enkephalin or beta-endorphin, they develop many of the symptoms of morphine addiction. Nonetheless, the recent discovery of the analgesic properties of neurotensin has aroused interest in its possible drug applications. According to Solomon Snyder, "Merck has made over 300 analogues of neurotensin."

Snyder personally believes that a different approach may ultimately prove more fruitful. "Making enkephalin analogues is just like making morphine," he says. "My own prejudice is that if we can find the enzyme in the brain that specifically destroys enkephalin and isolate it, then we could develop a drug that would inhibit this enzyme and thereby indirectly raise enkephalin levels. This would be a different way of juicing up the system, perhaps in a more gentle fashion than by having something that just mimics enkephalin.

Snyder's "prejudice" must have been well founded. Two months after our interview, this past September, Seymour Ehrenpreis of the Chicago Medical School reported the development of a drug, D-phenylalanine (DPA), that inhibits the enzyme that rapidly breaks down enkephalin. In 9 out of 11 chronic-pain patients, DPA brought about marked or complete relief from pain without causing sedation, a buildup of tolerance, or withdrawal symptoms after treatment was stopped. Furthermore, as in the fictional case of Barbara Loew, the patients who responded to DPA usually required only two days of treatment in order to obtain relief from pain for as long as a month. Ehrenpreis believes that this prolonged analgesia is the result of a long-term buildup of enkephalin levels in the brain. Laboratory tests with 200 mice have also found DPA to be nonaddictive, giving support to Snyder's contention that this method would prove to be a gentler way of "juicing up the system."

From these preliminary tests, DPA seems a likely candidate in the running for a miracle drug in the fight against pain. Indeed, for the nine patients who suffered from low back pain, arthritis, nerve injuries, and other debilitating forms of chronic pain, DPA has significantly changed their lives.

While DPA research continues, the medical community is watching warily to see if adverse reactions to the drug occur—especially those telltale signs of withdrawal. Past history of tampering with the brain's opiate system necessarily dictates a cautiously optimistic response to the new development. But today there is really good cause for optimism. The enormous growth in our understanding of the body's natural mechanism for coping with pain has not only revealed a scientific explanation behind esoteric methods for treating pain, but it has also suggested a cure that comes from within the body and the brain itself, especially through drugs that enhance the pain-suppression system without disrupting it to the point of addiction. Never before have the prospects of conquering man's oldest and most relentless enemy looked so promising.

CLONES VS. CANCER

By Owen Davies

Even a vampire settles for mere blood. Physicians at Boston's Sidney Farber Cancer Institute take the very marrow. But for children dying of leukemia, temporarily losing their blood-forming cells could be the best thing that ever happened to them. Removing their marrow is the first step in a startlingly effective new treatment for this fatal illness.

Traditional cancer treatments rely on radiation or harsh drugs to kill tumor cells. Most can be nearly as hard on the patient as on the cancer. The new procedures are based on antibodies, which are natural weapons the body uses to ward off illness.

Antibodies are the Sherlock Holmes of our defensive system. Whenever some foreign material enters the body—in an infection, say, or a transplant—antibodies ferret out the alien substances, called antigens. Then Scotland Yard, in the form of white blood cells and a material called complement, comes along to help finish them off. In the last five years or so, researchers have learned to arm antibodies against specific cancers. And they've discovered inexpensive ways to make copies — clones — of cells that produce these aggressive antibodies. Doctors call them monoclonal antibodies because the clones spring from a single (mono-) kind of cell. Many scientists think that these tiny, purebred, seemingly single-minded antibodies can put an end to the terror of cancer, possibly within the next ten years.

"What we do in leukemia is take out some of the patient's bone marrow and destroy the rest with radiation," explains Dr. Stuart Schlossman, head of the Boston project. Ordinarily this would kill the patient within a week because the marrow is the body's source of blood cells. But Dr. Schlossman's team treats the extracted marrow with complement and monoclonal antibodies that destroy the cancer, yet leave normal cells unharmed. Then doctors inject this marrow back into the patient. "When it works," Schlossman says, "this leaves the patient free of cancer cells — cured."

The key to this technique is to find the right antibody to attack the leukemia, then produce it in large amounts. It isn't easy. If antibodies are the immune system's Holmes, cancers are its Professor Moriarty, the villain too clever to be caught. Either tumor cells closely resemble healthy ones, or they exude some protective chemical that prevents the body from reacting to them. Other illnesses stimulate antibody production, but frequently cancer — even as a large, malignant lump — does not. Or when it does, the antibody concentration is too low to lock on to all of the intruder. So doctors have long sought a way to manufacture pure anitbody in large amounts — to amplify the human body's own weak defenses.

For a solution, researchers turned to a venerable laboratory ally: the white mouse. The procedure is almost cookbook simple. Scientists inject a bit of the human cancerous tumor into a mouse, whose system will react to any human cells as foreign. A day later the mouse is churning out antibodies as fast as it can. But it secretes tens of thousands or hundreds of thousands of different antibodies. A few combat the tumor. Most would attack the patient's normal tissue as well, if they were injected into the human. And the mouse produces too little antibody to cure even one patient.

So experimenters collect the antibody-producing cells from the mouse's spleen and fuse them with cells from a mouse cancer. Unlike normal tissue, cancers grow wildly, in the body or in the lab; this is what makes them so destructive. The hybrid cells produced by uniting spleen and tumor cells still secrete pure antibodies. Each cell's output is different. And because each cell is half-cancer, its descendants can be grown forever in laboratory flasks.

All that remains, then, is to screen each cell to find one whose antibody will attack the tumor in the human patient, but not normal tissue. A suitable cell can be mass-produced — cloned — as needed, and its antibody can be purified to get rid of contaminants from the mouse cancer that might themselves cause cancer in humans or — far more likely — an allergic reaction. The result is monoclonal antibody.

"Those are the big advantages: specificity and the unlimited quantity," says Dr. Jeffrey Schlom, of the National Cancer Institute (NCI). "People tried for decades to use natural mixtures of antibodies against cancer, and it never worked well. The key is to find the *right* antibody. Once you have it, making more is trivial. You just grow the cells. The amount of antibody you need to locate a tumor costs maybe a dollar. The drug companies are just going bananas."

Turned against leukemia, the antibodies developed at Farber have been spectacularly successful. Out of seven patients treated, only one has relapsed; the others have remained cancer-free for up to 18 months. In wide-scale use, antileukemia antibodies could save some 14,000 lives a year in the United States alone. And success to date is just a hint of what may come from antibody-based cancer therapies. Among the most important developments:

• One sixty-seven-year-old man seen at Stanford University suffered from a tumor that attacks antibody-producing cells. As recently as a year ago he would not have survived. To cure him, Dr. Ronald Levy, of the Stanford University Medical School, hatched an ingenious scheme. Like the cells from which it sprang, the cancer still produced antibodies. So Dr. Levy made a mouse antibody to attack the tumor-cell antibody, figuring that it would go straight to the tumor itself. Both standard cancer-fighting drugs and interferon had failed to halt the man's cancer. The monoclonal antibody stopped it cold.

• A test for several important cancers has been developed by researchers at Philadelphia's Wistar

Institute. The team has discovered a protein that seems to appear only in the blood of patients with pancreatic or colorectal cancer (of the colon or rectum). Monoclonal antibodies attach themselves to this protein even when it is present only in tiny quantities. By tracking the antibodies, doctors reveal not only the protein in the bloodstream but also the tumors, and with fantastic efficiency.

• Antibody-based scanners are allowing doctors to see tumors too small to appear on normal X rays. Labeled with radioactive atoms, monoclonal antibodies can zero in on a cancer within minutes, outlining it brightly on the screen of a computerized radiation detector—much like a CAT scanner—already used in major hospitals. According to Dr. Karl Erik Hellstrom, of Seattle's Fred Hutchinson Cancer Center, the technique can show hidden tumors only half an inch across.

• Ferritin, a protein found in normal cells, is produced by many tumors in large quantities. In normal tissue it aids in the use of iron; no one knows what it does for cancer cells. But in work by Dr. Stanley Order and his colleagues at John Hopkins School of Medicine, antibodies to it have shown signs of attacking cancers of the liver, lungs, and other organs.

Some of the most promising work with monoclonals has come in the field of lung cancer. "A truly usable antibody for lung carcinoma would be extremely valuable," notes Dr. Ingegerd Hellstrom, an immunologist who works with her husband, Karl, at Seattle's Hutchinson Center and holds a position as associate professor of medicine at the University of Washington. "There is so little to offer today."

A treatment for breast cancer is still far off, according to Dr. Schlom. But valuable diagnostic tests may already be here. "One very important use that's unique to breast cancer is a technique called lymphangeography," he says. "When a woman has a breast removed, the pathologist examines the lymph nodes near the armpit to find out whether she needs chemotherapy. If there is no sign of cancer in these nodes, the woman is sent home. Yet about a third of the women who are told they have no further tumor cells soon relapse.

"The trouble is that there is another set of lymph nodes under the chest wall. No one looks at them, because that would require major surgery. We can use isotope-labeled antibody to examine these nodes and perhaps catch tumors there."

But the real glamour in the antibody field is the hope that augmenting the patient's immune response will yield the cure for cancer. According to Dr. Order, there is good reason to hope. "We have tested antiferritin in twenty-five patients with a liver cancer so severe that half of all patients are dead three months after it is diagnosed," he says. "It takes nine months just to complete the treatment, and eleven patients who have done so show no sign of cancer. Antiferritin has also stopped Hodgkins disease and one form of lung cancer in four out of the five patients we've treated."

Another ingenious technique may also help prevent the rejection of transplanted organs. As a last resort in leukemia, doctors have often tried to replace the patient's bone marrow with normal marrow from a healthy donor. In most organ transplants, the body rejects the foreign tissue. But the transplanted marrow itself carries some of the equipment that does the rejecting; so in this case the transplant attacks its new body. The result is an often fatal illness known as graft-versus-host disease (GVH).

Dr. John Hansen, also of the Hutchinson Center, has prepared monoclonal antibodies against "T cells," the part of the marrow that attacks the host. Dr. Hansen used the preparation on patients whose GVH had already held out against the usual drug treatments designed to facilitate transplants. The antibody managed to halt the illness in 3 out of 12 patients. It wasn't a dramatic success, Hansen concedes, but it was enough to encourage further research. And there were no side effects.

Natural antibodies kill foreign cells both by attacking the cell wall directly and by calling in white blood cells that devour the invader. Researchers think they can make artificial antibodies far more lethal. Almost any poison that can be bound to antibodies, including the standard cancer drugs and radioisotopes, can be guided into tumor cells. One promising new candidate is ricin, a protein found in castor beans. Soviet secret police used it in London four years ago to eliminate a Bulgarian defector named Georgi Markov, Farber's Dr. Schlossman points out.

Researchers at the University of Texas Southwestern Health Center have already shown just how potent ricin-tagged antibodies can be. Working with mice, they have been testing a leukemia treatment similar to that used by Schlossman and his colleagues. The animals' marrow is removed, dosed with antibodies, and returned after a radiation treatment. But instead of using antibodies and complement, they are testing ricin-loaded antibodies. "The leukemia we use is extremely lethal," says Dr. Ellen Vitetta at the Dallas Center. "Yet about eighty-five percent of our test animals are permanently cured."

Before antibody-based treatments can be practical, some problems have to be solved. Antibodies now in use are made from mouse-spleen cells. After a few weeks of therapy, the patient's immune system recognizes the mouse protein as foreign and destroys the antibodies before they can attack the tumor. Scientists are now working to make antibodies from human cells. "'An easier way might be to switch animals," says Johns Hopkins's Stanley Order. "When the patient rejects mouse antibodies, go to rabbits or goats."

Another problem: It can be very difficult to find the right antigens to attack. Most antigens appear on normal cells as well as cancers. Stanford's Dr. Levy estimates that it takes six months to develop an antibody for use against cancer, and the process must be repeated for each patient.

Other researchers put their estimates far higher. Searching for antibodies that can be used against small-cell carcinoma of the lung, Dr. John Minna and colleagues at NCI screened about 20,000 antibodies; only 1 in 250 was worth a close look.

"I think the main problem is that many tumors are not uniform," says NCI's Dr. Schlom. "As the mass grows, many different types of cells appear. Some carry a given antigen; others right next to them do not. This is not true of leukemias or lymphomas, but for solid tumors it means that we may have to use several antibodies at once to get a cure." According to some recent experiments, killing only one or two of the cell types in a tumor may cause the others to grow rapidly.

And Dr. Karl Hellstrom points out that "probably no antigen is unique to tumors. They are simply much more abundant on the tumor cell." This is usually an important difference. If cancer cells are vastly more sensitive to a normal drug than healthy tissue is, doctors can dose the tumor fatally while leaving normal cells unharmed. With such potent toxins as ricin-loaded antibodies, however, *any* of the antigen on normal cells may attract a fatal dose of the poison, creating a situation comparable to death by "friendly fire."

"The question is whether ricin-carrying antibodies will kill even cells with just a few antigen molecules, and whether that causes trouble," Hellstrom says. "If they attack a cell that is common and not essential, that may not be a problem. But if the patient loses nerve cells, ricin may be too dangerous to use."

Some doctors are sure that ricin is too risky. "We've put in eighty years learning to use radiation safely, finding out how it will affect every tissue in the body," says Dr. Order. "Why do at all again for a new toxin?"

But Order has high confidence in other antibody therapies, and he flashes impatience at doubters. "The usual idea is that you cannot use an antibody against cancer that also acts against proteins found in normal cells. Yet ferritin, the antigen we attack, is found in many healthy parts of the body. People have driven me crazy over the fear that our antibody to it would kill normal tissue. For a long time the Food and Drug Administration would not approve our experiments because they thought I was dangerous. But we've given people large doses of antiferritin and never hurt anybody."

Even if fears continue to prove groundless, it is anybody's guess when patients outside these limited studies will receive antibody-based cancer treatments. "Logic has never been a virtue of the medical profession in general," Dr. Schlossman comments. "It can take years to prove to people that these results are not just luck. And you must understand that we get only the most difficult patients, the ones for whom everything else has failed. Nobody is going to start patients on these experimental therapies when there are already drugs for most of these diseases that work very well.

"Yet," he adds, "if a given antibody treatment does not pan out, it won't be because the principle is wrong. It will be because we are doing something wrong, and we can improve our current strategies. It will surprise me if antibody-based therapies are not in wide use within ten years."

Other researchers agree. Karl Hellstrom, seen by others as conservative in scientific matters, declares, "In ten or fifteen years these antibodies will revolutionize cancer treatment."

PART FOUR:
HERITAGE

THE GENE TRUST

By Kathleen and Sharon McAuliffe

From a chilled beaker, a scientist clad in white gently spools spaghettilike threads of DNA onto a glass rod. He is about to treat it with enzymes that will clip away all but a chosen gene, then insert it into the genetic material of bacterium called *Escherichia coli,* endowing the microbe with powers that nature never gave it.

Not long ago experiments with recombinant DNA stirred visions of strange, artificial diseases against which humanity would have no natural defense; such experiments provoked sharp controversy over whether scientists should be allowed to tamper with life itself. Today most of the fears have died down, and biotechnology is filling the heads of businessmen with visions of immense profits.

In the past ten years or so, dozens of new companies have begun to harness the life processes and put them to work in industry. Quietly, almost unnoticed in a world dazzled by innovative electronic products, these firms are fomenting a technological revolution that promises to shake the foundations of medicine, agriculture, food processing, energy production, and the chemical and pharmaceutical industries.

Already included among biotechnology's success stories are bacteria engineered to produce human insulin, drug-delivery systems that mimic the pancreas and other glands, microbial "miners" that leach valuable metals from ores, and novel pesticides that make insects their own worst enemies.

Yet, judging by the excitement within the business community, and the large capital investments these developing technologies have attracted, the most dramatic innovations are still to come.

"Commercial development of modern biology really only began in the early Seventies. By the mid-Nineties, certain applications will have proliferated in ways we just can't imagine," says Brook Byers, whose venture-capital firm, Kleiner, Perkins, Caufield and Byers, has put $1.5 million into two of California's pioneering biocompanies. One, Hybritech, has specialized in cloning specific antibodies that may someday destroy viruses and cancer cells. The other, Genentech, is working to synthesize recombinant microorganisms that will produce all the body's rare chemicals, from interferon to the opiatelike painkillers of the brain.

But few companies can outshine Cetus Corporation, in Berkeley, California, for sheer diversification. Chairman and co-founder Ronald Cape recalls, "When we started up in 1971, there was a tremendous amount of knowledge and discovery spanning a generation in molecular biology that had yet to find any practical applications. We knew that if we could tap only a small fraction of that potential, we'd be in business."

Cape and Peter Farley, president of Cetus, are among a rare breed of "hybrids"—a cross between serious scientist (Cape has a Ph. D. in biochemistry, Farley is a physician) and hard--headed, no-nonsense businessman (both hold M.B.A.s from prestigious universities). Joining forces with Donald Glaser, a 1960 Nobel Prize winner in physics, they were able to pool their special talents to become leading innovators of the new biology. Today Cetus has a market value of $75 million and counts some of the largest corporations in America among its shareholders.

Cetus, Genentech, and Hybritech all faced major problems in getting started.

"When we went out to sell our insights about molecular biology, we ran into brick walls," Cape says. "We were told we were dreamers. Now, eight years later, everybody's racing like hell to spend money in this area, and we're racing like hell to spend money faster to stay in the front line. It's difficult to believe how many people told us we didn't know what we were talking about."

One of Cetus's first goals is to develop a renewable energy source. With the world's oil supply dwindling rapidly, converting plant biomass into fuels and valuable chemicals is increasingly attractive. Sugarcane and sorghum, for example, trap up to 6 percent of the sun's energy that falls on their leaves. When these major food crops are harvested, however, millions of tons of bagasse, the leftover stalks, is thrown away. To convert this debris into ethanol for gasohol, Cetus intends to exploit the ravenous appetite of certain microorganisms.

"It's a coupling reaction," Cape explains. "The biomass becomes their food, and we use them as little chemical factories to convert it into alcohol."

The process now requires two kinds of microorganism: one that converts the cellulose in the biomass to glucose and another that turns the glucose into alcohol. Using recombinant-DNA technology, however, Cetus hopes to stitch the necessary genes from both microorganisms into one "superbug," which will perform the entire reaction.

MAN-MADE MICROBES

Although recombinant DNA enters into almost all research at Cetus, the company was not founded solely to exploit this technology. It was not until 1973, two years after Cetus was established, that Stanford University's Dr. Stanley Cohen and others began developing means to transplant genes from one microorganism to another. The original plan was to harness the astounding versatility of natural microbes, which had been all but ignored by commercial enterprises. The unexpected advent of recombinant-DNA techniques simply speeded their progress. Suddenly scientists could endow their "bugs" with entirely new abilities, tailoring them to fulfill industry's needs.

Within Cetus's eight buildings, dozens of breeds of bugs are rapidly multiplying. They may well become an indispensable work force in the future. Huge amounts of single-celled protein may be continuously harvested in one lab to provide livestock feed for countries that lack soybeans. Another microorganism can convert ethylene to ethylene glycol, a principal component of antifreeze. Recombinant-DNA technology may induce still other microbes to produce a sticky, jellylike substance that will coax oil in abandoned wells through the surrounding rock and up to the surface. (After a well has gone "dry," close to 60 percent of the oil may still remain in the ground.)

"We've devoted ourselves to trying to do things for industry that industry hasn't yet been doing for itself," says Cape, whose microbial army is set to make a wide range of chemical products — from plastics to fertilizers — now derived from oil and gasoline. Biological production would save energy, according to Cape, and would reduce pollution and lower the operating costs of traditional chemical synthesis.

One naturally occurring bacterium has already proved its cost-effectiveness in extracting valuable metals from low-grade or inaccessible ores. Mining companies in Canada, Australia, and the United States are investigating the possibility of using microbial processes to supplant conventional mining methods altogether.

Microbes hold even brighter promise for medicine. The body's most potent chemicals exist in minute quantities and are extremely difficult to extract and purify. The scarcity and exorbitant cost of these substances prevent their use by doctors.

Interferon, for example, has been available only to a handful of medical researchers. Even if it should prove to be a powerful weapon against cancer, as researchers suspect, who will benefit when its current price is $22 billion a pound? However, Cape is confident that genetically engineered microbes will solve this problem — and in the not-too-distant future. "I think we'll be getting useful amounts of interferon into people's hands within the next two or three years, at a much lower price than they have to pay now," he reports.

DNA FACTORIES

Although gene grafting was first carried out between breeds of bacteria, it soon proved possible between widely different organisms. When mammalian genes are spliced into bacterial hosts, these microscopic factories can be tricked into producing large quantities of natural body substances — hormones, enzymes, and antibodies — which are difficult or impossible to obtain synthetically.

For the pharmaceutical industry, this development marks the beginning of a new era, and Cetus is not alone in seeking to cash in on it. In South San Francisco, California, Genentech has announced the first synthesis of human hormones in recombinant bugs. A much smaller company than Cetus, Genentech has as its exclusive goal the commercial development of recombinant DNA. Starting with only $1 million in venture capital, president Robert Swanson was able to launch into business quickly by hiring researchers in universities and private institutions to take on projects for Genentech in their own laboratories. While hunting down scientists willing to do commercial work, Swanson met Herb Boyer, a biologist who has made some of the most important discoveries in recombinant-DNA research. The two readily formed a partnership.

The big payoff came scarcely a year later, when Genentech scientists, working with the City of Hope Medical Center in Los Angeles and Boyer's laboratory at the University of California, succeeded in coaxing a strain of *E. coli* to produce the brain hormone somatostatin. Genentech has patented the process, which is expected to lower somatostatin's price from $300,000 a gram to $300 a gram.

Following this breakthrough, Genentech announced two more genetic engineering feats: microbial production of insulin and, more recently, growth hormone, used to treat pituitary dwarfism in children.

From a commercial standpoint, insulin so far is Genentech's most spectacular success. The American insulin market is estimated at $137 million, 80 percent of which is controlled by the pharmaceutical house Eli Lilly. Genentech has signed a contract with Lilly to market human insulin. Most insulin is extracted from the pancreas of pigs and cattle, but one diabetic in 20 is allergic to the animal hormone. This new source will save the life of such patients.

While genetic engineers have been refining their methods in the last decade, other scientists have been finding new body chemicals that might revolutionize medical therapy. Particularly exciting are enkephalin and beta endorphin, opiate-like substances produced by the brain that emerged as powerful pain suppressants during recent clinical trials. Like interferon, these intriguing compounds have become a target for recombinant-DNA researchers at Cetus, Genentech, and elsewhere.

In the last year or so at least three more companies have entered the race to exploit genetic engineering: Bethesda Research Laboratory and Genex, both in Maryland, and Biogen, in Luxembourg. In addition, some larger and longer-established companies are now setting up their own research and development programs.

It will probably be several years before the products of genetic engineering reach the market. Once a discovery is patented, its manufacturer must test the product rigorously to meet the standards laid down by government watchdog agencies. In evaluating the first drugs ever obtained from recombinant bugs, the Food and Drug Administration is likely to be exceptionally cautious. This could mean five to ten years of testing and up to $50 million in costs before the product goes on the commercial market.

Yet industry on the whole has not tried to resist these precautions. Although most scientists now believe the potential hazards of recombinant-

DNA research were grossly overestimated, public alarm over the safety of such research is a good enough reason for industry to regulate itself voluntarily. According to the Pharmaceutical Manufacturers Association, its half-dozen member firms engaged in recombinant-DNA work have all agreed to abide by the National Institutes of Health guidelines, which now apply only to non-industrial research. The guidelines stipulate, among other things, that dangerous recombinant-DNA experiments be carried out in containment areas, the so-called P-4 facilities.

"Most people don't realize how conservative business is," says Byers, whose venture-capital firm has been closely watching ongoing developments. "The fear of liability is enormous. It could ruin a company overnight. So it is perfectly rational for businessmen to spend the money to ensure maximum safety."

GENE GAMBLING

Another way to mix the genes of different microorganisms — cell fusion — so far has escaped the controversy whirling around recombinant-DNA research. Cell fusion mates the unmatable, combining the cells of organisms that don't ordinarily breed. Cetus and some of the larger pharmaceutical companies are experimenting with the new technique.

"There are times when you simply want to play a crap game with the genes without being as directed as recombinant DNA is," Cape says. "In other words, just push all the genes in two different cells together and sort out what happens. It's a lot more efficient toward certain goals." Research contracts prohibited him from revealing what projects are under way at Cetus, but it was cell fusion that allowed Otis Godfrey, of Eli Lilly, to fuse two antibiotic-producing microorganisms last year. The result was a hybrid capable of synthesizing a new antibiotic unlike those of either parent strain.

Cell fusion is still in its infancy, but at least one innovation based on it has already been heralded as an advance no less important than recombinant-DNA technology. In 1975 Dr. Cesar Milstein and his colleagues at the Medical Research Council laboratory, in Cambridge, England, stumbled on a way to fuse a myeloma (skin cancer cell) with an antibody-producing white corpuscle. The result, called a hybridoma, began to turn out pure specific antibodies. Moreover, the relentless growth of the myeloma gave the hybrid cells virtual immortality.

Until Dr. Milstein's discovery, the only way to obtain antibodies was to trigger their production in laboratory animals. But harvesting antibodies from the animal's blood serum produces a mixture of antibodies in which some are more specifically directed against the intruder than others. Milstein's technique, however, enables scientists to separate out the hybridoma whose antibodies can distinguish the intruder from all other cells and then to mass-produce them by cloning. His research offers the long-sought "magic bullet" that will destroy viruses and cancer cells without damaging healthy tissue — the major drawback to the "shotgun" therapies now employed.

Hybritech, a year-old firm in La Jolla, California, is already producing antibodies using hybridoma. According to president Howard E. Greene, its early goal is to provide antibodies for clinical diagnostic tests, with a potential U. S. market of about $200 million a year. The company's first product, now being sold for experimental use, is a series of antibodies for detecting hepatitis B. Also under development are antibodies that will aid in the diagnosis of such hard-to-pin-down diseases as heart attack and cancer of the prostate and colon.

Diagnostic materials are less strictly regulated than drugs, and Hybritech plans to consolidate its earnings from test kits before expanding into therapeutics in about five years. The hope for the future is to inject antibodies directly into the body to cure numerous diseases ranging from hepatitis to influenza to cancer.

"Many scientists view cancer as occurring because the immune system can't recognize malignant cells," Greene says. "In other words, certain individuals may fail to generate antibodies against cancer." If hybridomas can be created from the white blood cells of people who can produce such antibodies, Greene says, "You ought to have one of the best possible forms of cancer therapy imaginable — one that's based on our natural defense mechanism."

NATURE'S BLUEPRINT

Genetic engineering and cell fusion are not all there is to the biotechnology revolution. The new life manipulators are developing many other exciting medical and industrial techniques modeled on nature's blueprint. At Alza Corporation, in Palo Alto, California, researchers are designing sophisticated drug-delivery systems that will help doctors use human insulin, the brain's opiates, and other body chemicals.

These substances are extremely powerful and, at high concentrations, can be toxic, even fatal. The problem is that after an injection or tablet, drug levels in the patient's body peak rapidly, then dwindle. This fluctuation is a major cause of many dangerous drug side effects.

To prevent this, Alza is mimicking the endocrine system, where each gland secretes its hormones at a controlled rate, without unwanted side effects. Devices now under development deliver medication slowly and only where it's needed — in the eye, uterus, or circulatory system, for example. One mimics the pancreas, continuously releasing tiny amounts of insulin that can be fine-tuned to meet the diabetic's individual needs.

Alza recently received permission to market a three-year birth-control system in Mexico. Placed in the uterus, the device continuously releases progesterone, a natural birth-control hormone. Because the progesterone is released slowly, the device avoids the unwanted side effects of the Pill.

One of the most promising drug-delivery systems being tested at Alza is an "osmotic minipump," a capsulelike unit that can be implanted, injected, or swallowed. Activated by water, it can dispense several drugs at varying rates, either simultaneously or in succession. Eventually physicians will be able to make up a whole two week drug program and install it in the patient. Such complex and reliable drug schedules will make many common medications much more effective.

"We are also talking of a sampling device, a sucking device," reports Dr. Alejandro Zaffaroni, the company's founder. Instead of dispensing medication, it would take repeated blood samples for up to two weeks or so, preserve them, and send them into a machine for analysis.

"I believe it will give a whole new dimension to medicine," Dr. Zaffaroni says. "Instead of analyzing just one blood or urine sample gathered during a physical exam, you'll get a complete picture of how the patient functions in his daily life. A person might, for example, seem to have normal blood pressure in the doctor's office, yet have episodes of very high blood pressure. That patient is at risk and should be considered for treatment."

Another Zaffaroni enterprise, Dynapol, is working to eliminate the possible hazards of food additives. In light of the recent saccharin scare and the dwindling list of food dyes now approved by the FDA, Dynapol set out to develop dyes, sweeteners, and preservatives that would not pass through the wall of the intestine and into the body.

Dynapol has found a way to leash small food-additive molecules to larger, indigestible polymers. The resulting macromolecules, unaffected by storage, cooking, and the digestive processes, will enter the market in 1981.

PETER PAN HORMONE

At Zoecon Corporation, another research program has led to the world's first commercial insect-growth regulator. Known as methoprene, it interrupts an insect's normal life cycle by blocking maturation. This regulator, a synthetic imitation of a natural insect hormone, is a most effective pesticide.

According to John Diekman, vice-president in charge of research and development at Zoecon, "Insects go through dramatic metamorphoses from wormlike larvae to hard-cased pupae and then on to the adult stage, with full wings. Zoecon and other university researchers set out to isolate the growth chemical turned on and off by the brain during this process.

The natural hormone had problems. It was not powerful or selective enough, it was too expensive, and because it was natural, it couldn't be patented. Zoecon overcame all these drawbacks by synthesizing a chemical that mimics it.

Methoprene works by keeping insects that are problems in the adult stage, such as mosquitoes and the hornfly (a major cattle pest), from fully maturing. It is completely unlike conventional pesticides. "We call them insect-growth regulators," Diekman explains, "because it's not a hard pesticide. If you spray it on a bug, the bug does not immediately drop dead. The methoprene affects the insect's hormone balance, and when the bug is ready to mature, it can't, and it dies."

The insect-growth regulator is so unusual that Zoecon was one of the first firms Chinese scientists requested to visit when Henry Kissinger's exchange programs began. "I'm sure Kissinger and Nixon had no idea what the heck an insect-growth regulator was," Diekman comments.

Methoprene is now the safest pesticide available. It is biodegradable and nontoxic to other organisms. Indeed, it is so safe that it is fed directly to cattle. When consumed, it passes through the animal's digestive tract and comes out in the manure, where the flies breed. "Instead of going around the King Ranch and trying to spray every manure pile," Diekman says, "you can use the cattle as your applicators, and the maggots die in the manure."

Ironically, the product's safety became a real headache for Zoecon when the firm set out to obtain regulatory approval. The Environmental Protection Agency demands to know what happens if you overdose an animal on a pesticide. Zoecon's problem: Methoprene is so safe that an animal can't overdose.

Zoecon is trying to develop a juvenile hormone antagonist, methoprene's mirror image. Instead of retarding growth, this antagonist would accelerate it, to turning insects that, as juveniles, cause tremendous crop damage prematurely into pupae.

Diekman says, "We don't think the Environmental Protection Agency creates incentives for the type of novel research we've done here, and we've been vocal about this. Dr. Carl Djerassi, our chairman, has met with all the important regulatory agencies. But we're tired of fighting. We'll continue to increase our budget for insect control, but we're faced with long lead times, heavy investment, and a moderate success rate." So Zoecon has decided to branch out into other biotechnologies.

Zoecon's long-term plan is to explore plant genetics. Using genetic engineering, Zoecon hopes to produce better plants, strains that are more disease and insect resistant, with higher yields. Researchers will attempt to do in the laboratory what takes years, or may even be impossible, using classical plant-breeding techniques.

THINKING BIG

The history of biotechnology, though short, is repeating the pattern of innovation in this country. Over and over again the trendsetters have been fledgling firms willing to risk their money. Dr. Cape says, "The large companies, with very few exceptions, have been caught flat-footed by these rapid developments in biology. The same was true for the semiconductor field.

"When new technologies come along, the people who should throw themselves in, hook, line, and sinker, don't. You would have imagined that Bell Laboratories, General Electric, and RCA would have jumped at the opportunities presented by transistor and semiconductor technology to become the big powers in the industry today. They're not. None of them are. Texas Instruments is, Motorola is, Fairchild is, Intel is, National Semiconductors is. They're the upstarts that came in to fill the vacuum."

Will Cetus, Genentech, Zoecon, and the other pioneers of biotechnology become the corporate giants of tomorrow? It's still too early to say. But the industry as a whole is entering a period of massive growth. Even its most optimistic proponents have been awestruck by how rapidly their dreams have been transformed into financially rewarding undertakings. Few people in industry remain unconvinced that there is big money to be made.

Biology's leap from academia to the commercial world may have come later than that of either physics or chemistry, but its impact on our lives promises to be just as far-reaching. In the next 20 years it will dramatically change everything from the practice of medicine to the world's supply of food and energy. We have only begun to unlock biology's secrets—the technology of life itself.

ANTICIPATION

By Dr. Bernard Dixon

Hemophilia and sickle-cell anemia are clear-cut examples of genetic disorders, but what about duodenal ulcers, fibrositis, or skin cancer? As our concept of exactly what constitutes a hereditary disorder broadens, genetic counseling will no longer be limited to those who are concerned about their offspring having a birth defect. In the future, six-month-old babies will routinely have their white blood cells analyzed, and parents will be presented with an outline of specific diseases the infant will be susceptible to over the entire course of his or her life.

Such information leads to obvious practical action. Parents of a child who is vulnerable to skin cancer, for example, may decide to leave sunny California and make their home amid a less beneficent climate on the East Coast. An adolescent who is likely to fall victim to painful fibrositis in middle age may decide *not* to pursue an athletic career that would only aggravate the condition. Ulcer proneness may influence an individual's choice of diet or even his or her livelihood.

The idea of being able to assess disease susceptibility later in life is a startling one. Knowing *what* they might get, and *when*, could lead to radical changes in people's careers, life-styles, and expectations.

No standardized method of plotting a personal index of probabilities has yet been adopted, but one approach hinges on the discovery of HLA antigens. These first came to light because they affect the acceptance or rejection of tissue grafts. Just as blood groups determine the types of blood that can be transfused from one person to another, so HLA antigens must be matched if a kidney or other organ is to be successfully transplanted. These antigens occur on white blood cells and tissues, and their myriad subdivisions constitute a "chemical fingerprint."

As immunologists began analyzing HLA antigens, it was soon apparent that antigen patterns provided telltale signs of our predisposition to different diseases. Rheumatoid arthritis, multiple sclerosis, psoriasis, and coeliac disease are among the conditions known to be influenced by them. And the list is growing steadily. HLA antigens might radically transform genetic counseling as we now know it.

The profession's rapid advancement is also due to parallel findings that have emerged from a closely related field. While one group of researchers have focused on HLA antigens or cell-surface markers, still others have probed inside the cell to study chromosome abnormalities. Such a technique is used by cytologists to disqualify female Olympic athletes whose cells show signs of illicit intersexing, but its greatest potential may be to highlight disease proneness. One example appears in the recently published annual report of the U.K. Medical Research Council. It raises the prospect of distinguishing between tobacco smokers who are vulnerable to lung cancer and those who are comparatively resistant.

The research is being done by Professor H. J. Evans at the Clinical and Population Cytogenetics Unit, in Edinburgh. So far he has shown that some cigarette smokers have significantly more chromosome defects in one sort of white cell, compared with nonsmokers. Moreover, a particular chemical in smoke, even in vanishingly tiny amounts, causes these cells to mutate. Studies are now under way to compare the response of cells from lung-tumor patients and those from healthy controls. Evans's next step is to learn whether this approach can be extended to identify sensitive individuals.

There are further indications that such an exercise may be rewarding. Already one cell defect — the so-called Philadelphia chromosome in some types of leukemia — has been linked unambiguously with cancer. More recent reports suggest that subtle chromosome abnormalities are also associated with kidney carcinoma and with several other forms of leukemia.

The impact of these converging fields of reasearch is immediately apparent: Tomorrow's medics will be able to give us uncannily precise information about our future medical profile. Whether we will take heed of that advice is, of course, an entirely different question.

SPARE GENES

By Yvonne Baskin

The conveyor belts of the Central London Hatchery and Conditioning Centre move slowly through the crimson twilight of the Brave New World, carrying human embryos toward their "decanting" stage. Into various bottles go typhoid inoculants to prepare some embryos for work in the tropics. Heat conditioning will make some hate the cold. Constant motion improves the sense of balance of future rocket pilots. Oxygen and alcohol levels adjust intelligence.

Half a century after Aldous Huxley's grim prophecies, human intelligence, behavior, and desires still lie beyond our control. But mankind is on the brink of being able to alter his genetic programming with more precision and more selectivity than Huxley ever imagined.

The dramatic impact will come first in medicine, opening up possibilities for correcting tiny chemical quirks in our genes that can cripple our minds and bodies, lower our defenses, and sentence us to early death. More than 3,000 currently incurable hereditary diseases will come under attack from pioneers on this dramatic new frontier—gene therapy.

Twice in the past ten-year period physician-researchers have transferred foreign genetic material into young girls doomed to retardation or early death by errors in a single gene. Neither attempt brought any improvement in the patients, and heavy criticism speedily ended both projects. However, even critics who called these experiments premature predict that more attempts will be made within two to five years to transfer "good" genes into human beings. By the end of the decade scientists may be able to offer treatment for any of a dozen defective or missing genes.

Diagnosis will move ahead even more quickly than therapy. Researchers armed with new, automated tools of genetic engineering — robots manipulating molecules to make components of artificial genes — will isolate the biochemical mistakes responsible for hundreds of inherited disorders. Within the next ten years machines may routinely scan the genes of a fetal cell for abnormal "fingerprints," which signal problems ranging from color blindness to cystic fibrosis. Heart disease, cancer, alcoholism, aging, and other undesirable conditions or afflictions may also one day be ameliorated by advances in gene therapy. Research now in progress in labs across the country may determine the specific genetic components that are "triggered" by cholesterol, cosmic rays, viruses, a whiff of solvent, or one nitrite-filled hot dog too many.

And what about intelligence, emotion, behavior, character? Are they, as sociobiologists contend, at least partially programmed by our genes? Will the knowledge gained in medical therapy inevitably lead some people to try to tamper with the nature of man, either by manipulating genes or by aborting for traits we feel are undesirable?

"I've argued for four or five years now that at some point the sociobiologists and the genetic engineers are going to converge," says Sheldon Krimsky, a Tufts University philosopher of science who serves as a member of the federal Recombinant DNA Advisory Committee. "The sociobiologists believe you can find genes for altruism or sexism, and so someone will undoubtedly look for them."

But W. French Anderson, of the National Institutes of Health (NIH)—like many molecular biologists—is not ready to worry about such speculation. "The scenarios that envision great changes taking place in humans—that might be something to worry about fifty years from now, or even twenty-five years from now, but certainly not in the next decade," he says. "People who want to influence complicated phenomena, like behavior, would have better success with drugs," he adds.

"Until somebody has isolated a gene that has anything at all to do with intelligence or personality or behavior, there really isn't any room for speculation," Anderson says.

Our genes, 50,000 to 100,000 of them—we don't yet know how many—make up our mission-control team. Strung out at their posts along 23 pairs of threadlike chromosomes in the nucleus of the cell, the genes guide the transformation of a single fertilized ovum into the 100 trillion specialized cells that an adult human being possesses. Each gene, composed of DNA, has a single duty, to provide a "blueprint" for the manufacture of one protein. The blueprints are elaborate: If all the genetic material—DNA—in just one human cell were removed and unraveled, it would stretch to about six feet in length.

In every cell of an organism, the gene team is the same. But the mission varies. Nerve cells don't make insulin, and skin cells don't make blood proteins. In any nucleus, some genes lie dormant; others may be shifting to new posts; and the rest are busy directing the production of their proteins.

Every member of the team is so crucial to the mission that even a minute aberration can be disastrous. An errant gene may ignore directions and produce too much of its protein, or make it at the wrong time, or botch the order and turn out an abnormal product. Or it may fail to produce anything at all. Then body secretions may thicken and clog the lungs; red blood cells may become distorted and pile up like a logjam in the capillaries; nerves may degenerate. Bones and facial features may become deformed. Toxic wastes may build up while any one of 100 necessary chemical reactions fails to occur.

Repairing a gene is still in the realm of science fiction. But adding genes to dilute out defective genes in individual cells has become a realizable goal.

The critical steps in such therapy are as complicated as finding and blunting a million needles in a million haystacks. After discovering which gene is malfunctioning, researchers have to isolate it, reproduce millions of copies of a working replacement gene, insert the new genes into appropriate cells, and see to it that the new genes produce what they're supposed to produce in a controlled way.

Not one of these steps was possible 12 years ago, when biochemist and physician Stanfield Rogers made a unique attempt to treat patients by using foreign genetic material. Rogers, who had been studying the cells of rabbits for more than 15 years, heard about the affliction of two little German girls. He thought he could see a connection between their cases and his research; he flew to Cologne to see them.

"The older child—about five years old then—was having a really tough time walking across the room," he recalls. "Both parents had to hold a hand to help her. She was obviously retarded and suffered convulsions. The two-year-old was in pretty good shape. It didn't appear that anything was wrong with her."

But the blood of the younger child—and of a

third sister, born a year later—showed the same previously unknown abnormality found in their eldest sister. The blood of all three contained unusually high amounts of an amino acid called arginine, one of the building blocks the body uses to construct protein. An enzyme, arginase, is supposed to keep blood arginine levels under control, breaking down the excess. But the gene for arginase was apparently missing or defective in the girls.

This problem indirectly caused another: The oldest girl's brain damage probably resulted from ammonia intoxication, Rogers thinks. "Ammonia is handled by being converted to arginine. Having so much arginine probably inhibits the synthesis of more, and you get a buildup of ammonia."

As head of a cancer-research program at Oak Ridge National Laboratory, in Tennessee, during the 1950's, Rogers had been using Shope papilloma virus—which causes benign, wartlike tumors in rabbits—to study how viruses turn normal cells into tumor cells. Rogers observed that rabbits infected with the virus had low blood arginine levels. He found evidence that the virus carried a gene for arginase. Another surprising finding came a few years later: Half the laboratory workers handling the virus had low blood arginine levels like the rabbits. Until then it had been assumed the virus did not infect man. Could the virus provide the girls with a gene for an enzyme to protect them against ammonia poisoning?

Bravely, Rogers set up a clinical trial—the first of its kind—to find out. He obtained some of the girls' cells, infected them in a lab dish with virus, and found they contained the same protective arginase discovered in the rabbits. He put a vial of highly purified virus on ice and took it to Germany with him. "In the first injections, we didn't know how much to give," he says. "We gave a dose about the same amount we'd give a rabbit."

Rogers sent more virus over when the third girl was born. Then came a serious setback. "When they sent me the virus to test, it had gone to hell," he says. "When I tested it, there was no activity whatever." No matter what the reason was—too small a dose, an inactive virus—the girls' blood arginine levels didn't change.

Anderson, at the National Institutes of Health, believes Rogers "did everything possible to make sure the experiment was as correct, ethical, legal, and appropriate as possible, and he was very open about it." But a tidal wave of professional criticism swept over him. His funding withered away. He turned to plant genetics.

Rogers, now past sixty and recovering from a stroke suffered several years ago, expresses no bitterness about the criticism and the career setback. "It never did bother me much, because I knew that philosophically we had to do it," he says in his Southern drawl. "These kids who have these diseases, they're in miserable shape. If we can do anything to stop their disease, I think we must do it."

The public took little notice of the work Rogers was doing. Genetic engineering was not yet the stuff of headlines. But by the middle of the 1970s the public began to pay attention.

By then scientists had learned how to isolate single genes and use new techniques to produce unlimited clones, or copies, of them. They cut open rings of bacterial DNA, called plasmids, with chemical "scissors" and spliced foreign genes into the circle. The plasmid then infected the bacteria, carrying with it the foreign gene. The dividing bacteria became a kind of factory producing millions of copies a day of the plasmid and the foreign genes. Then the genes could be recovered from the bacteria and purified.

As purified genes became available through these techniques of recombinant DNA, the next step was to try to insert them into cells. Success came in 1977 to Richard Axel and his colleagues at Columbia College of Physicians and Surgeons, in New York City. The procedure—used widely today—turned out to be simple kitchen chemistry.

The researcher draws a measured amount of a clear, watery solution of purified genes into a pipette and releases it into a plastic tube containig another clear liquid, a calcium phosphate solution. He waits 30 minutes or so until the liquid becomes slightly cloudy. This indicates that calcium is precipitating out of solution with the genes.

A few drops of the precipitate are added to human or other mammalian cells, growing in a watery nutrient medium in a petri dish. For some reason yet unknown, the gene is taken into the nucleus and integrated with the cell's own DNA, in a process called transformation.

In a nation where *recombinant DNA* had become a household word, this first gene-transfer work hardly seized the public imagination. The get-rich-quick-in-biology fever had largely eclipsed the first fears of "Satan bugs," clones of Hitler, and plant/people monsters. Public excitement had focused on the simpler and more profitable feat of putting genes into bacteria for mass production of interferon, insulin, and other pharmaceuticals. But the headlines for gene transfer into animal cells weren't far off. Within two years of the Columbia experiments came the first transfer of isolated genes into living animals and, a breathtakingly short time later, into man.

One of the most tragic aspects of cancer is that

any treatment for it is often as devastating as the disease itself. Powerful cell-killing drugs, such as methotrexate, used to fight tumors, also damage normal cells, especially vulnerable bone marrow.

Methotrexate kills cells by inhibiting an enzyme, needed in the formation of other essential chemicals. But certain tumor cells eventually develop a resistance to methotrexate by producing multiple copies of the gene for this enzyme. This platoon of genes can turn out more enzyme than the drug can block, and the cell survives. This is, of course, an undesirable trait in cancer cells. But if this ability could be transferred to healthy cells, doctors could give larger doses of methotrexate to cancer patients and their bone marrow would still survive.

In April 1980 nationally known blood specialist Martin Cline announced his University of California at Los Angeles team had transferred this genetic protection to the bone marrow of living mice.

Cline had taken bone-marrow cells from mice and incubated them with the protective genes by using the method developed in Axel's lab. Cline and his colleagues injected all the cells back into mice whose marrow had been destroyed by radiation.

Then the team gave daily doses of methotrexate to the rodents. The cell-killing drug prevented proliferation of the transplanted marrow cells that hadn't taken up the protective genes. The resistant cells flourished. Defended by injections of genes, the mice became inured to the adverse effects of the drug.

Cline announced then that in "three to five years" such a system might be tested in human cancer patients to allow them to tolerate higher, more potent doses of antitumor drugs. Not known as a man to hang back and wait for the crowd, he wasn't planning to wait half a decade before trying gene transfer in humans. The first disease targeted for gene treatment, though, was not cancer. It was an agonizingly painful blood disorder.

All of the 100 trillion cells in the body depend on the protein hemoglobin in the red blood cells to deliver the oxygen they need to function. The wear and tear of surging through the blood vessels limits the life of a red cell to about four months. Consequently bone-marrow cells are kept busy turning out new red cells at a rate of about 2.5 million a second.

When the genes responsible for making the components of hemoglobin can't keep pace, or when they deliver defective parts, or when they don't work at all, the results can be devastating blood diseases. In sickle-cell disease, a chronic anemia that afflicts about 50,000 blacks in the United States, the red cells are rigid and distorted, making it hard for them to squeeze through tiny capillaries. When they get stuck and block blood flow, the result is severely painful "sickle-cell crisis," often followed by death.

Among the peoples of the Mediterranean, the Middle East, and the Far East, another life-threatening group of hemoglobin defects—the thalassemias—pass from generation to generation. In persons afflicted with beta zero thalassemia, one of the proteins needed to build normal hemoglobin is not supplied because of a defective gene. Red blood cells, made by the marrow, are brittle and shatter easily.

In the spring of 1980, as Cline was proclaiming the first gene transfers into animals, a woman in Jerusalem was piling up losses in her 21-year battle with beta zero thalassemia. Her body, in a desperate attempt to make enough replacements for her fragile red blood cells, produced so much marrow that her bones became deformed and her face was distorted with oversized "gargoyle" features. She had suffered numerous disfiguring fractures, which left her with a limp and made walking a painful task.

The billions of red blood cells shattering throughout her body over the years had left behind a deadly accumulation of iron, which was crippling her heart. She had been hospitalized frequently for chronic heart failure. The blood transfusions she needed to stay alive only made the iron overload worse. Intelligent and aware of her condition, she also knew that few victims of the disease live past their twenties.

Cline had been thinking about a way to attack the hemoglobin diseases long before he met the young woman in Jerusalem: Why not remove bone-marrow cells from the patient, insert good genes, and put the cells back in the patients?

An aggressive and self-confident physician, Cline, forty-seven, was already a recognized world authority on bone-marrow cells. He was a relative newcomer to molecular biology. Nevertheless, he decided the time was ripe for trying the gene transfer.

But there was a major hitch. No one had ever got the genes to work properly in cultured cells. Cline went on to the next experimental step. He tried putting the human genes into mouse bone-marrow cells and transplanting these cells into mice. The genes didn't work there, either.

Still, in the spring of 1979 Cline asked UCLA review committees for permission to try gene-transfer therapy in sickle-cell-anemia patients. He also sought permission from hospitals in Italy and Israel to try the therapy in thalassemia patients.

A few months after the announcement of his methotrexate work in mice, Cline flew to Naples to meet with colleagues at the University Polyclinic. He took along samples of human genes for a component of hemoglobin. And he carried the genes with him when he flew on to Hadassah Hospital, in Jerusalem.

At 7 A.M., on July 10, 1980, Hadassah officials notified Cline that permission for human work had been granted. Cline lost no time. By 9 A.M. the twenty-one-year-old victim who was to be the world's first gene-therapy patient had arrived at the hospital.

Two hours later she was given local anesthesia. Her hipbone was pierced with a long needle, and 15 milliliters of marrow (only a fraction of the 10 liters in the body) and blood that was circulating through it were drawn out.

The marrow-and-blood mixture was placed in a dish, and a precipitate of calcium phosphate with genes was added.

Five hours after it had been removed, the blood-and-marrow mixture was injected into a vein—standard procedure in marrow transplants. The cells—400 million of them, perhaps 5,000 carrying new genes—circulated in the blood and eventually homed in the marrow.

Within the week, Cline flew back to Naples and performed the same procedure on a sixteen-year-old girl from Turin. Unlike the Israeli patient, the Italian teenager had no gross bone deformities. But she had been dependent on transfusions since early childhood, and iron overload was already harming her heart.

In Los Angeles that same week, convinced that more animal work was needed, the UCLA committee turned down Cline's application to transfer genes into sickle-cell patients.

When news of the human experiments broke in October 1980, a furor erupted in the scientific community. With unaccustomed ferocity, researchers throughout the United States publicly accused Cline of leaping blindly and abandoning good scientific judgment in an effort to be first.

"He was hoping against hope the genes would work in humans when they never had in other animals or cultured cells," one molecular biologist says. "That's nonsense. It's like pouring water into your car and hoping against hope it'll work like gasoline."

A committee of the NIH later found Cline guilty of violating several federal guidelines, saying he should have obtained permission from UCLA for the work he did abroad. UCLA accepted his resignation as chief of hematology-oncology. By the end of 1981 he remained a tenured professor, although he lost $190,000 — about half — of his federal grants.

As for the two patients, all Cline will say now is that they are still "clinically okay." But reports from Italy and Israel indicate blood samples from both girls haven't changed. If the new genes were working, some normal hemoglobin should be present.

Were there any risks in the experiment? Could a new gene bump other normal genes or control mechanisms out of place on a chromosome? Could an improperly regulated gene produce too much of a protein product or wander from the target cell into other cells where it didn't belong?

"There are always those possibilities," Cline says. "It may well be that when one begins to introduce large amounts of genetic information, with some low but real frequency you will turn genes on that you don't want to turn on." But in the first experiments on patients who already have fatal diseases, he doesn't see the potential risks as serious problems.

Disheartened by the affair and somewhat rueful because he didn't follow the rules with more patience, Cline still defends the experiments and their timing. Most of his critics were lab scientists, not clinicians, he says, and such people don't see the plight of dying patients.

"In the initiation of most treatment for lethal diseases like cancer, a good deal less is known than was known at the time these studies were begun," he says.

He believes someone else would have tried the replacement therapy in a year or two or three, at most, if he hadn't. "Probably more intelligently than I did, more circumspectly," he admits. "The field has gone fast, extremely fast. And, even though studies on humans are temporarily suspended, clearly it's going to be a matter of only a few years.

"I think most people agree that gene therapy is a real possibility in the future. No one I know of has said, 'No, you won't be able to replace genes.' The criticism has come in the timing and in how much we must know before we proceed."

There is almost universal agreement among scientists that one thing we must know before applying these techniques to humans again is how to get transferred genes to work right. Two or three years ago, buoyed by the rapid advance in gene isolation, cloning, and transfer, scientists—apparently including Cline—were optimistic they they would quickly learn to control genes. But it has turned out to be, as California Institute of Technology molecular biologist Leroy Hood puts it, "a very nontrivial problem."

Anderson sees at least three problems to separate and solve before natural gene control is understood. First, bits of DNA that switch genes on and off, like a light switch placed far from the lamp it regulates, may lie far upstream on the chromosome from the genes they affect. Even if a section of DNA with both the gene and its control element on it can be snipped off and isolated, it might take too long to clone with current techniques.

The two other problems arise in the cloning. A dividing bacterium — foster home for nurturing genes — may not be able to equip the gene copies with some specific, important modification they would get if they were being produced naturally in a developing embryo. Finally, packaging and position on the chromosomal thread may be important. A "naked" gene, isolated and cloned, may lack the element of control that comes from the coiling of DNA in the nucleus.

Some genes are easy to turn on. The human-growth-hormone gene, for example, can be inserted into various kinds of cells. No matter which cell they're in, hormones can control them, Axel says. His lab has also achieved success with "heat-shock genes" taken from fruit flies. These dormant genes in fruit flies are activated when the temperature rises 12 degrees above normal. Inserted into mammalian cells, these fly genes still go into action when the temperature rises.

Another gene that scientists believe may have a simple on-off regulation is one that directs production of an enzyme called HPRT (hypoxanthine guanine phosphoribosyl transferase). A deficiency in this enzyme causes a horrible form of cerebral palsy called Lesch-Nyhan syndrome. Children afflicted with this disease, if not restrained, will chew off their lips and fingers and bite others who come near them. Many labs are working to isolate the gene.

Researchers are also looking for more efficient ways to get new genes into cells, though none of the methods now being studied appear suitable for immediate use in humans.

One way involves loading genes aboard viruses,

simple and tiny microorganisms that invade and take over cells. Nobel Prize-winner Paul Berg, of Stanford, and many other scientists are exploiting the ability of tumor viruses to break through cell walls and command the production of more viruses. Whole tumor viruses are not suitable for human experiments, although stripped-down viruses are now being developed that will not kill the infected cell or turn it cancerous when the virus carries genes into the invaded cell.

Another gene-transport system is deceptively simple: Squirt genes in through the cell wall by using a tiny glass needle. Anderson's team has used this process to insert new genes directly into the nucleus of a single mammalian cell. Other researchers have made rapid advances by using this technique to inject genes into a fertilized egg. Jon Gordon and Frank Ruddle, of Yale, are nurturing a third generation of mice that carry human interferon genes, although the genes are not working to produce interferon.

The researchers allow mice to mate normally, then a few hours later remove the fertilized eggs from the female. Looking through a microscope, the scientist pierces an egg with a hollow glass needle only a few ten-thousandths of a millimeter in diameter and releases a spurt of genes.

The work is challenging. Sometimes the cells swell and burst. "On our best days we probably kill a quarter of the cells just by putting the needle in," Gordon says.

The researchers can inject from 50 to 100 eggs a day and surgically implant the survivors into female mice. Half the embryos may survive to birth, and one embryo may actually carry the foreign genes. Gordon says. "Although it sounds tedious and difficult, it's a fairly high-efficiency procedure," he notes.

Thomas Wagner, of Ohio University, and Peter Hoppe, of Jackson Laboratory, in Maine, advanced the process one step further when they used the same technique to transfer rabbit genes for hemoglobin into mice. Not only have the rabbit genes been passed on to a second generation of mice, but some of the mice are actually making the rabbit protein.

Now that human eggs can be fertilized in a test tube and be reimplanted in women who produce healthy babies, microinjection techniques open up the possibility of gene therapy at the embryo level. But Gordon isn't sure we'd ever want to use it.

"If you have prenatal diagnosis so sophisticated that you can identify a bad genetic makeup at the one-cell stage, then you can simply not reimplant that embryo," bypassing therapy, he says.

If injection therapy were used, would a gene inserted into the embryo begin to work in every cell of the adult? "It could be a very serious problem if a person were making hemoglobin in his brain or liver or kidney," Gordon says.

"We can treat some human diseases with this technology without ever microinjecting a human egg," he adds. Studies of gene function in animals may lead us to better solutions for disease and defects than are now imaginable.

Cline agrees that microinjection may not be ready for use in human embryos "for decades and decades, if ever." But therapy of the type he tried in order to cure diseases caused by single genes is not far off, he predicts.

"There's five or six years of doing this type of work ahead of us to perfect the technology that can get the genes in consistently, and in the right place, and get them expressed at reasonable levels," Cline says. "But I would guess that within the next five years or so the technique should be widely applied to man."

Automation is speeding the process of identifying which defective proteins are associated with genetic disorders and then tracking them back to the genes.

In Leroy Hood's lab, at Caltech, sit two automated biochemistry sets the size of washing machines. One is a sequencer. It can take a few millionths of a gram of protein, chemically snip off each amino acid like beads from a necklace, and identify them by liquid chromatography. The sequence of amino acids spells out the DNA code of the gene that made it.

Armed with the code, Hood can punch it into the keyboard of the other instrument, the gene synthesizer. A microprocessor takes over, opening and closing valves, systematically releasing multicolored reagents, solvents, and chemicals onto a small disc, where a portion of an artificial gene is assembled piece by piece. The end product is a fine white powder, dehydrated genetic material.

The powder is like a copy of a piece in a jigsaw puzzle: It can be used to search for the original piece. Radioactively labeled, the synthetic gene material probes the DNA isolated from a cell, then links up with the natural gene from which it was copied.

"I would predict in five years that we'll have DNA probes for one hundred or two hundred human genes, many of which are involved in genetic diseases," Hood says.

And he foresees even more sophisticated instruments that might scan fetal genes for defects. Fetal cells removed from the uterus now by amniocentesis can be examined only under the microscope for gross abnormalities in the chromosomes, or extra chromosomes that signal diseases such as Down's syndrome.

Someday the DNA from these cells may be broken down into thousands of fragments and be run out on a gel that separates them according to size, Hood says. Then a defective gene responsible for sickle-cell of some other disease could be radioactively labeled and added so that a possible match among the fetal genes might be discovered.

"There are probably thirty-five hundred human genetic diseases that have been defined, and far fewer than two hundred can be diagnosed by amniocentesis if we use current techniques," he says. "The hope is that with recombinant-DNA techniques we may be able to look at far and away the vast majority of these."

With anything beyond single-gene traits or functions the timetable for gene therapy becomes fuzzy. "As soon as you begin to deal with complex multigene systems, the problems multiply that much more," Cline says. "You have to identify all the genes and have them arranged in some way so that they can be controlled coordinately."

But the possible limits of the field don't daunt zealous researchers. "I think recombinant DNA is going to be the biggest thing for the next ten to fifteen years in medicine, period," Hood says. "In diagnosis, in therapy, in the potential for understanding at a fundamental level the nature of disease."

The only uncertain thing is the timetable, Hood suspects. "Clear technical problems remain," he says, "but if you take the broader view there's no question that we'll solve them all."

For some observers, the ethical and social questions loom larger than any technical problems still to be faced. Mistakes and misuse seem inevitable, says Theodore Friedmann, of the University of California at San Diego. But he and other scientists don't want to see the pursuit of knowledge hampered by questions about how wisely society will apply the fruits of research.

"This work is not being carried out by megalomaniacs or crazy people who are doing it just because it can be done," he says. "The exciting thing now is that, for the first time, one is imagining treating metabolic diseases where the defect is instead of treating only the symptoms."

But how far should "therapy" go? "Should we try to eliminate genetic diseases?" Sheldon Krimsky, at Tufts University, asks. "Are we obligated to do this? Who should make the decisions?"

Should therapy be limited to the correction of defects in individuals, or should we attempt to improve the germ cells of people who carry hereditary diseases? "Do we want to improve the species? As we learn more about the impact of the environment on genes and about which genetic sequences are associated with longer life spans or a more effective immune system, opportunities will arise to play this kind of genetic-engineering game on a fertilized egg," Krimsky says.

"I'm concerned about the programming of the fertilized egg or the newborn with particular characteristics. I worry about the onset of a genetic aristocracy," he says. "It'll be, 'You mean to tell me your child does not have genetically engineered into him or her the genes for—' and you name it.

"Beyond that, it's the idea that scientists and medical people possess the wisdom to determine what the prototype of a human being is," Krimsky says. "It's that area that people are not talking about now because they're really not at that stage. But with the idea of mapping the human genome, it won't be that long, twenty or thirty years, before we begin correlating genetic sequences with a propensity toward certain diseases."

It is a well-meaning but misguided use of science that presents the real danger, Krimsky and others believe. Who wouldn't want a perfect baby? But scientists today are universally opposed to tampering with the human embryo.

News articles glibly refer to a future when we will program our cattle to put all their energy into producing milk and we'll engineer our crops to survive on salt water. Will we use our burgeoning knowledge to enhance the individual? Or will we use it to make individuals, like cattle and plants, to suit society's needs?

From the herds of identical semimoron Epsilons to Alphas with carefully programmed intelligence, most of the characters in Huxley's vision were content. The world was at peace. Rage and passion were tamed. Aging and disease were banished. Fantasies and fears, dreams and ambitions — all flattened to a frightening monotony. It is good to remember that the Brave New World was born of benevolent intentions.

PREDESTINATIONS

By David Rorvik

Five hundred years hence, Aldous Huxley forecast in his novel *Brave New World*, a "biological revolution" will invest a scientific elite with awesome powers of "genetic predestination." That revolution is already upon us. Historians will look back on the tag end of the twentieth century as a turning point in the ascent of man, auguring the new era of "participatory evolution."

The late Nobelist Dr. Edward L. Tatum has called the growing ability of *Homo sapiens* to engineer the genetic future of the species "the most astounding prospect so far suggested by science." Caltech biologist Robert L. Sinsheimer terms it "one of the most important concepts to arise in the history of mankind." He adds, "For the first time a living creature understands its origins and can undertake to design its future."

Not everyone is sanguine about what all this portends for mankind. To some, genetic engineering is a monstrous affront to God and nature, a forbidden act of cosmic masturbation: man with his hands down his genes, fiddling with himself. One does not have to turn to the fundamentalists to hear this attitude. Even a "liberal" panjandrum like Norman Mailer laments that the bioengineers have now "bored through the outer cores of pornography" to arrive at the very "rim of conception." They are, he shudders, "Looking to operate on the Lord."

Some of the bioengineers themselves have serious qualms about man's headlong rush into creation, fearing that we now have the ability to create but not the wisdom to know what, when, or whether to create. "Our ignorance is profound," declares Nobel Prize winner George Wald, urging a moratorium on much of the current gene tinkering.

"Have we the right," asks Columbia University biochemist Erwin Chargaff, "to counteract, irreversibly, the evolutionary wisdom of millions of years in order to satisfy the ambition and the curiosity of a few scientists?"

The trouble is, it is no longer merely a few scientists. It is a multitude of scientists, and it is business—big business. Genetic engineering is being touted, with increasing persuasiveness, as "the next big growth industry," potentially bigger than the semiconductor industry, which is sponsoring its own revolution in another dimension. "The new IBMs are in the making right now," says an executive of one of the fledgling bioengineering outfits.

The biological revolution is proceeding along

two parallel fronts. The first is genetic engineering—"recombinant DNA," "gene splicing," and so on; the other is "gametic engineering," the *in vitro* manipulation of germ cells, including such phenomena as test-tube babies and cloning. Several human test-tube babies are already among us—the result of eggs that were fertilized in laboratory dishes and then reimplanted in the women from whom they were first obtained. These forerunners of the test-tube generation will soon be joined by brothers and sisters who will be the products of more exotic genetic engineering. Embryo transplants will allow women who do not produce viable eggs of their own to bear a child. They will also permit "normal" women to have children of their own without the inconvenience or risks of pregnancy.

Human-egg banks are already joining human-sperm banks. Soon they will merge to form human-embryo banks. Indeed, there are gametic enterprises gestating in the cradles of corporations whose studies have convinced them that it may be both feasible and profitable to offer life for sale in frozen pellets. Animal-embryo banking is already a substantial business. There is no doubt it will work as well with human embryos. One Indian test-tube baby, before implantation, had been deep-frozen until the prospective mother's reproductive cycle reached greatest receptivity.

It was Dr. Hermann Muller, winner of the Nobel Prize in medicine, who suggested many years ago that embryos grown from gametes contributed by only the "best" of us be frozen and made

227

available to inferior mortals, in an effort to "improve" the human gene pool. Recently it was revealed that a sperm bank, modeled along the lines proposed by Dr. Muller, has been established: utilizing the sperm of Nobel laureates. The only donor so far willing to identify himself is Dr. William Shockley, the Nobelist who had previously "fathered" the transistor.

Cloning, the duplication of an organism from a single body cell, has now been achieved, not only in reptiles but also in mammals. Many physicians have proclaimed that mammalian cloning is still years, and probably decades, away. They were undoubtedly somewhat embarrassed when Dr. Karl Illmensee and his colleagues at Geneva University, in Switzerland, announced this spring that they had cloned several mice, the cells of which are, in many respects as difficult to deal with as human cells. Dr. Landrum Shettles, a pioneering reproductive biologist, reported last year in the *American Journal of Obstetrics and Gynecology* that he had succeeded in microsurgically transferring the nuclei of human spermatogonial cells (sperm precursors that still possess a full set of chromosomes, like any other body cell, as opposed to the half set contained in the mature germ cells) into human eggs with their nuclei removed. In three cases the clone showed healthy development to the stage where an embryo normally attaches itself to the womb lining. "There was every indication," Dr. Shettles reported, "that each specimen was developing normally and could readily have been transferred *in uterum*." The foremost obstacles to cloning humans, he now concludes, are "social rather than scientific."

Plant cloning is already a flourishing enterprise. Livestock cloning is expected to become a multimillion-dollar business in the next few decades. Soviet scientists, eager to increase milk and meat production, claim the ability to replicate large animals. Humans, too, are bound to avail themselves of cloning technology.

Some may want to use human cloning not only to foster fertility but to guarantee a child of one sex or the other and, perhaps, to produce an ego-gratifying "chip off the old block," literally the "spitting image" of the old man (or woman, as the case may be). Individuals unhappy with what they see in the mirror may recruit the genetic material of others. Columbia University sociologist Amitai Etzioni argues that a black market in body cells, bought or "ripped off" by wholesalers, will arise in our lifetime, making it possible for couples with cash in hand to give birth to carbon copies of film idols, sports figures, popular leaders, and so on. Using cell-freezing techniques, nostalgia buffs may be able to birth anew the heroes of yesteryear.

Such abuses will pose no great threat to society as a whole, but they will complicate the lives of those human copies, who will have to struggle harder than ever to develop unique identities. Much more controversial is the prospect of keeping "decerebrated doubles," their cloned copies, as living but mindless repositories of "spare parts" that could be transplanted, as needed, without risk of rejection. With a "parts replace ment" program like this, individuals might live decades longer.

All sorts of macabre possibilities loom ahead. With the advent of ectogenesis—complete test-tube fertilization, gestation, and birth—we will have easy access to the developing fetus, to correct defects and, if we desire, to alter developments. Such a technique might produce endless batches of happily disposed, defect-free, blue-eyed, blond-haired, pink-skinned monotonies—if we wished. Researchers have already sustained mammalian test-tube life beyond the stage at which major organs begin to form and function.

There are people willing and eager to meddle in gametic predestination, some by trying to dictate who may reproduce with whom, others through direct genetic intervention. Muller's program of "germinal choice," recently revived, is but one example. Several scientists have suggested that prospective parents be required to pass tests to determine their genetic suitability for parenthood. Nobelist Sir Francis Crick has gone further, asserting, "No newborn infant should be declared human until it has passed certain tests regarding its genetic endowment . . . If it fails these tests, it forfeits the right to live."

One cannot discount the possibility, however repugnant, that committees of creation may one day oversee human evolution. Technology available to us today permits us to join the cells of different mammalian embryos, the offspring having not the normal two parents but as many as six. Hundreds of multiparented mice have been thus created. Given the undying impulse of the eugenicists to "improve" the human race, the time may arrive when children will be "constructed by committee," perhaps under computer guidance indicating which genetic traits in aggregate would create a person of "optimal" specifications.

The implications of genetic tailoring are even more unsettling. Beginning in the 1970s, scientists discovered a method of transplanting genes into bacteria that reproduce themselves through simple division, creating precise duplicates of themselves each time they divide. Employing this method, one can make billions of copies of the transplanted gene in a matter of hours. Through these novel techniques it is possible to analyze gene function and to engineer bacteria that, thanks to the "foreign" genetic instructions that have been spliced into them, will churn out large quantities of enzymes, hormones, antibiotics, and other valuable substances in short supply. Insulin, human-growth hormone, and the antiviral agent interferon have already been produced in this inexpensive and time-saving manner.

Further refinements of these methods may enable men to isolate, rearrange, and even create entirely new genes for specific purposes, introducing them into individuals deficient in them or targeted for "improvement." Just as we confer remarkable abilities upon bacteria today, inducing them to perform functions as alien as it would be for a milkweed suddenly to start yielding cow's milk, so we may endow ourselves with unimagined capabilities, creating not merely a different man but a different species of man.

Genetic engineering, even when it does not impinge directly upon human genes, may have an enormous impact upon human evolution. Man-made DNA "chimeras" that now exist or that could soon be made will "eat" oil spills, convert waste into useful energy, and allow plants to obtain nitrogen directly from the atmosphere, eliminating the need for artificial, possibly harmful, fertilizers. All such developments are bound to help shape our evolutionary destiny, perhaps for the good.

But critics of gene-splicing work charge that there is also a potential for disaster. Noting that genetic instructions for the production of cancer and other dread diseases are being spliced into bacteria with an affinity for the human body, these critics raise the specter of a new killer bug being accidentally unleashed on a vulnerable population. Thus, the debate about genetic engineering focuses primarily on what regulations and safeguards must govern this work. These fears may have some merit, but they have been exaggerated.

Accidents are not the real danger. Willful abuse is, and in the long run the most insidious danger of all is well-meaning misuse. Though some of the bioengineers sincerely insist that gene splicing is "inherently benign," just as another group of researchers earlier promoted the dream of "the peaceful atom," there is little doubt that gene splicing is being used to produce new bioweapons that could someday make the old germ warfare seem tame by comparison. Assurances that we are protected from such perils by existing treaties will help only the naive to sleep soundly.

Despite assertions by President Nixon in 1969 that we were retiring our bioweapons unilaterally, the CIA is suspected in 1971 to have introduced a virus into Cuba that forced the slaughter of half a million swine, temporarily dislocating the Cuban economy. In 1972 the U.S. Army undertook an ambitious study of various "inherited blood characteristics" and their geographic distribution. A seemingly related Pentagon study focused on the blood proteins of "different Asian peoples." Papers published in *Military Review* and elsewhere have revealed a military interest in ethnic weapons, calling attention to ethnic/racial genetic peculiarities that might be taken advantage of in "recombinant" warfare. The enzymatic "eccentricities " of blacks, Asians, and Semitic peoples have attracted special interest, both in this country and in the Soviet Union. Two molecular biologists from the USSR who now work at the Weizmann Institute, in Israel, assert that Soviet researchers are aggressively investigating genetic vulnerabilities. Terrorists, too, can be expected to take note.

The line between outright abuse and well-meaning misuse blurs abruptly in those instances where the armed forces, insurance companies, manufacturers, and others are investigating genetic factors in an effort to separate "bad" risks from "good" ones. The DuPont Company, for example, now routinely screens black job applicants in search of the sickle-cell trait. The screening, some charge, is used to divert blacks from certain jobs; DuPont responds that it is all part of an innovative effort to keep "susceptible" individuals away from potentially toxic materials in the workplace. MIT molecular biologist Jonathan King, an outspoken critic of genetic engineering, states flatly that "DuPont's position is scientific racism. People are not going to get sick because they are hypersusceptible; they are going to get sick because they are being poisoned." A study funded by the U. S. government has sought genetic traits that dispose one toward antisocial or violent behavior. The ostensible goal is to weed out these traits in a program of genetic "prior restraint."

These and other developments portend an invasion of privacy that may ultimately provide "scientific" bases for discrimination, alienation, and exclusion more powerful than any yet experienced. Genetic screening, for all its potentially positive contributions, may eventually serve as a means of declaring certain "genetic types" dangerous, useless, inefficient, or obsolete. We have already subverted the rich diversity of nature in our successful efforts to create, through similar genetic intervention, vast monocultures of "miracle crops" that have proved vulnerable to outbreaks of unexpected or unfamiliar diseases. We may likewise be in peril of producing equally vulnerable human monocultures.

Instead of addressing the causes of violence, we are now attempting to eradicate our ability to be violent. Instead of improving our diet and cleaning up our environment as a way to fight cancer and other "diseases of progress," we are hunting for a recombinant "magic bullet" that will cure, rather than prevent, these diseases and that will allow us to go on polluting ourselves and our world. There are recombinant bugs in the works that will let us digest plant proteins, turning us into grass eaters and thereby solving the world'ss food-shortage problem (at least for a while), encouraging us to keep on overpopulating. And if the crowding causes stress, the stress can undoubtedly be dealt with through a little genetic surgery.

These new technologies, I fear, will not make man more noble, more compassionate, more aware of his own diverse mystery, but rather more malleable, more tolerant of social and evironmental decay. The "super race" whose advent so many have feared will not be the forced irrational product of a mad dictator's dreams but the cost-analyzed, market-tested, pragmatic product of profit-oriented scientist-businessmen. Blue eyes and blond hair won't be a fraction as important as the ability to endure stenches, stress, verminous food, crowding, industrial pollution, boredom, and depersonalization.

The New Man will be remarkably stable, non-violent, defect-free, well adjusted, "responsible," and like the New Bread that is already with us, bland, short on real nourishment, processed, refined, whitened, artificially preserved and fortified, and baked to absolute uniformity. And no one will doubt him when he asserts he's happy.

PART FIVE:
MIND

LANGUAGE, EMOTION AND DISEASE

By Wallace Ellerbroek, M. D.

Some years ago, when I was a little younger but just as peculiar, I was a general surgeon more interested in why people got sick than in cutting them—and equally interested in why they got well. Eventually, I decided that if I were to get any of my crazy ideas accepted, I'd have to become a psychiatrist. So I started hunting for a psychiatry residency. I was interviewed by one eminent gentleman and incidently expressed my belief that anger and depression were important mechanisms in the induction of cancer. He sneered, not very politely, and said, "Every weekend we get at least a dozen nuts in the emergency room who have figured out what causes cancer." I asked, "What do they say?" His reply, which I treasure, was, "We ignore them . . . we have better things to do."

Better things to do? Yes, I suppose so. From

his point of view we already know that cancer is caused by this, that, and the other thing. The list grows daily—just watch your newspaper.

Although I will concede that constant exposure to soot does relate to carcinoma of the scrotum among chimney sweeps in England, I have difficulty accepting the idea that everything I like is carcinogenic. I am told, in numerous scientific announcements, that maraschino cherries, barbecued meats, the water I drink, and the air I breathe are all going to lay me low. And that's not all. Eggs, sugar, milk, cream, butter (my wife and I probably eat several tons of these deadly items per year, to the accompaniment of shrieks from our friends) are all denigrated by the utmost authorities. Leaving the worst for last, tobacco, the sin of sins, as well as coffee, the mainstays of my existence and functioning—well, they say you would be safer sitting all day playing Russian roulette with a forty-five!

This all sounds very sensible, but it nonetheless leaves me entirely dissatisfied. Some people smoke and get lung cancer; lots of people smoke and don't get lung cancer. My questions remain unanswered: why *do* people get sick? And why do some stay sick? And why do people get well, and if they don't, why not?

Are these impossible questions? At the moment, given the available models, it would appear so. Physicians, of course, have all the answers unless you look closely. They have names for all the known diseases—sometimes, lots of names—and people do feel some relief when given a name for what is bothering them. Afflicted individuals pestiferously return to the doctor or chiropractor or, lately, to an infinite variety of gurus and complain that they feel no better.

We have doctors whose model for "diseases" are due, they say, to "real" organic causes. We also have the psychosomaticists, most of whom give a fairly clear message that, basically, it is all in your head. Sandwiched in between is a new breed of patient, semi-antiestablishment, who enjoys health food a lot. This group is uncomfortable with partisans of either of the former approaches and is searching out "alternative treatment modes." In former days, people who employed such therapies were called quacks, but now they seem to be practicing holistic medicine, acupuncture, acupressure, transcendental meditation, faith healing, and who knows what else. For those who want something to smear on, shoot up, or ingest, we have royal queen bee jelly, Laetrile, Krebiozen, and other varieties of rather more concrete treatments.

The really weird thing is that *all* of these work — sometimes, somehow, and to variable degrees. But people still get sick. As soon as we stamp out one disease, a worse one appears. Sometimes without stamping one out, a new one starts in: it almost seems as if we *must* have disease. We have to get sick, one way or another, in spite of, and more frequently now *because of,* scientific advances.

"Iatrogenic" is an increasingly popular word for the trouble you get *after* you go the the doctor. There are even people who are hideously ill yet — to paraphrase Shakespeare — prefer to keep those ills they have than fly to medical management they know not of. Are there medical advances? Yes, of course, but if you add them all up, particularly here in scientific America, we humans should not be having high blood pressure, obesity, coronary artery disease, and on and on. I won't even mention the unconquerable head colds, sinusitis, and, in the young, ear infections, tonsillitis, acne vulgaris, and much, much more.

Yet all the same, the clues abound. Once in a great while you encounter an individual who has managed to live to an advanced age, who is not sure what doctors are for, since he or she never goes to see one, and who dies — usually while asleep — without assistance from contemporary diagnosis or scalpels. Others, it seems, are the opposite, always having something wrong somewhere. They look at you blankly when asked when they last were well. Most people are somewhere between these two extremes, having alternating periods of health and sickness over the years, the finale being some type of unsuccessful major medical ritual. Finally, there are the so-called cancer miracles, which do actually happen, however rarely.

All this seemed clear to me in 1960 or thereabouts. I imagined that thoughts, language, and emotions had a good deal to do with illness. (For this I was considered quite disturbed by many of my associates.) The crux of the matter was that each patient, with all his or her problems, *should have exactly those problems*. The more deeply I went into that person's behavior, thinking, and lifestyle, the more sense it made. Most particularly, it seemed that unhappiness, of whatever type, was an integral part of getting sick.

I recall a charming young woman afflicted with a relatively common though obscure condition called "idiopathic cervical adenitis." This means that she had swollen glands in her neck that were tender and bothersome; no one could figure out why. She had seen dentists, throat specialists, and internists to no avail. I was treating her for something else but became interested in her neck difficulties, and we talked a good bit. She was a lonely girl, rather prudish, slightly overreligious, and very inexperienced in the ways of the world. She found most males overly aggressive in sexual matters, so never dated. Suddenly, while she was still my patient, a man in her office started to show considerable interest in her. Within a few weeks she was a changed girl — sparkling, alert, wide-eyed. And, fascinating to me, the chronically swollen nodes in her neck completely disappeared. This lasted six weeks; then she found out that he was married, happily so, with a gaggle of children. Literally within a matter of days, the nodes returned, accompanied by their associated miseries and distress.

To my amazement, I was soon able to find similar factors in every patient I saw. Some cases, as the one above, were obvious. Others were extremely obscure, requiring long periods of observation. Many patients totally denied carefully concealed emotional pains, while others were completely unaware that they *were* unhappy, feeling this to be their "normal" state. I gradually learned ways to get through to them and in the process learned how devious the human mind can be.

At one point I began to realize that the puzzles of human illness were *not* insoluble. I gave occasional lectures (and was considered something of a quack), but mainly I kept working with patients and studying in all directions. I learned of Darwin's 23-year silence and so kept silent — for the most part. The exceptions were my frequent letters to the editor and book reviews, each with one or two of my own ideas tucked in: a comment on wedding-ring dermatitis, a brief discussion of the emotional feedback of shoulder posture, a hint that schizophrenia might be caused by disturbed thinking (instead of being the cause of disturbed thinking), and so on.

But the climate gradually changed, and now I no longer wish to avoid open publication. So, let's state a few basic definitions and postulates and then proceed:

• There is no such thing as a fact: any verbal statement is an *opinion,* no matter how labeled. For example, any statement can be called either an opinion or a fact. If you call it an opinion, you bear in mind the possibility of error. If you call it a fact, you are neurotically expressing a belief that the statement is gold-plated, never to be questioned, and, more important, you are turning off your thinking machine as to that item.

• Objective knowledge is a myth: all "knowledge," being based on biases in "perception" and "cognition," is subjective and emotionally determined.

• There are only two emotions, like and dislike:

all others are compounds of one of these plus a personally formulated comment about "reality" (e. g. "lonely" = I am all alone now + I do not like being alone).

• Anger and depression are *not* separate emotions. Anger is: "Reality, as I seem to perceive it, does not match my fantasy of how it ought to be, but I think there is something I can do about it." Depression is the same, except . . . "but there is nothing I can do about it."

• (This one is critical.) Negative emotions are associated with unnecessary disturbances of bodily mechanisms, proportional to the duration and intensity of the negative emotional state. Such reactions are *not* limited to a particular organ. All bodily organs and cells express their response to such brain states in various ways. If you are angry or depressed about your job, your stomach acids will either go up or down; your blood pressure will go up or down; your glands will increase or decrease their functioning, etc.

Consider the concept of "stress." There are, from my point of view, two reactions to stress. If it makes you miserable, your body will have all kinds of deleterious reactions. But if the stress is enjoyable—pursuing a not-too-willing member of the opposite sex, for example—the stress will make both you and your body function better than ever, up to the limits Mother Nature herself has installed.

Is there, then, a significant possibility that anger and depression, rather than being normal and necessary concomitants of human existence, are the long-sought variable factors in the development of *all* human diseases, both "mental" and "physical"?

This idea, bizarre as it sounds, has been for me of enormous clinical utility, and I do believe it has enormous potential for the welfare of everyone. It means that you can do something to try to avoid getting sick. It also means that if you are sick, there is something you can do to promote your recovery. And, of particular interest to the medical profession, it eliminates the idea that there are "untreatable" diseases and affords new approaches to the major human scourges — cancer, coronary artery disease, and hypertension, to name a few.

This entire subject is, of course, incredibly complex: if my ideas seem simplistic, they are not — I have seen them work when all else failed. But before going on, I would like to insert a bit of personal history. In medical school, where I was able to listen to what I was told — and to repeat it back in test situations — they told me: "Measles is caused by a virus, and that's a fact." In my head I recorded, "*They say* measles is caused by a virus, and that is an opinion." Some of their "facts" seemed potentially useful, so I decided to hang on to all of them in case they came in handy. Some did; a lot didn't. So I became a doctor and later a surgeon and later a psychiatrist, but always with a head full of questions.

I became extensively concerned with the state of mind of my patients, both before and after surgery. At the same time, I became deliberately introspective, trying to look into my own head to see what was going on and how it worked. The net result of all this was an enormously changed state of mind on my part concerning the nature of my patients and their illnesses and how to care for them. I found that scientific medicine alone was not enough, and that my intense emotional involvement with the patient was part of the treatment. Further, I found that *anything* I did to make the patient *feel* better helped him to get better.

I continued to practice "good" medicine by eliminating treatments or medications that in some way made the patient feel worse. I also added anything that had a definite "positive placebo" effect. Critical to all this was my belief that I *could* help the patient, no matter what the diagnosis. Equally critical was my ability to make the patient feel the same thing. The results? My patients did better, recovered sooner, and had fewer complications. Even people hopelessly ill or dying showed definite improvement in the quality of their remaining existence.

Now let's start over and try to answer a few of those impossibly difficult questions.

Why do people get sick? It is *not* due to "physical" or "mental" factors but to the *sum* of all factors: physical, mental, emotional, and environmental, past and present. Careful observation, however, suggests that negative emotional states of some type are almost always present and contributory. Further, it is my opinion that what actually happens to people is not as important in producing illness as what they *think* happened is. In other words, if something bad happens, you don't *have* to get sick if you can avoid getting miserable about the situation.

Why do people get what *they get when they get it?* This is the problem of psychosomatic specificity (e. g. what all the people with certain diseases have in common). If you consider *everything* that has happened to an individual since conception (or before), everything others have said to him or her, every thought he or she has ever had, plus everything that has been happening in the universe during the corresponding time, it becomes obvious that each person should, at any instant in time, have exactly what he or she does have. And when you look closely, you do discover that people with similar diseases have similar patterns, most particularly in their thinking.

The American Cancer Society provided me with an excellent example of the disadvantages of "normal" thinking. In an ad, underneath a series of photographs showing a little boy and girl holding hands, the caption read: "Little children shouldn't get leukemia." According to me, that message has a number of less than desirable effects: it makes you angry or depressed, and more seriously, it does not lead to open thinking. Try this instead: "Since certain children do get leukemia, if we understood all the factors, it would become obvious that those children *should* have gotten leukemia."

This phrase opens your mind to an infinity of questions, a few of which just might be important in seeing what the processes actually are. The problem is, of course, in the word "should." In the first case, it means "it would be nicer if," but it is expressed in a psychotic manner, e. g.

contrary *to reality.* In the second case, it means "it is appropriate that" and is more in accord with so-called reality as we perceive it.

Does this mean that all diseases are mental? No. I say that mind processes (which means the functioning of the total brain in the body) are indeed part of, but only part of, getting sick or recovering.

Then how we think does contribute to getting sick or well? Exactly! And this brings up the other problem, equally complex, of just how our language affects our perceptions and behaviors. I will only indicate here that: (a) language is full of traps, (b) there is no single *right* word to apply to anything or any process, and (c) each word you use as a label for something makes you see it in an entirely different way. Say "I am free" and mean it. Say "I am a slave" and mean it. Then alternate — and watch your feelings.

Having arrived at that point, perhaps we can now start talking about the diseases so prevalent in our day, and what, perhaps, each of us can do to avoid getting sick; or if sick, what we can do to restore ourselves to health.

Obviously, we cannot discuss here all the major diseases so I picked one that is now practically epidemic and truly a major public health problem: high blood pressure. It wrecks hearts, kidneys, and other things and leads to one of the most tragic of human conditions, a stroke. Worse, the incidence is currently increasingly at a horrendous rate. A few cases are due to certain peculiar "physical" lesions, but the vast majority are what is called "ideopathic" or "essential" hypertension, which means the cause is unknown. Some doctors feel that it is inherited or "genetic" (loosely translated, "good luck, buddy"). Others blame diet, salt, your job, your wife or husband, etc., etc., *ad infinitum.*

A few researchers, particularly those into biofeedback, currently hold that anger is a cause. They are close, but not close enough. One person came much closer, back in 1952. While studying the attitudes of patients with a variety of diseases at New York Hospital-Cornell Medical Center, Dr. David T. Graham found that those with hypertension "felt that they constantly had to be ready for anything." (The reference is: Psychosom Med 14:243-251, 1952.) This was a genuine, gold-plated clue, though his work was put down, ignored, and largely forgotten . . . but in a few moments you will understand the significance of his finding.

Remember, I called all diseases "behaviors," in other words, things that people do, and hypothesized that *if* something was wrong, then there was something that the person was unhappy about. When I found a patient with elevated blood pressure (140/90 mm/Hg or more). I said to myself not "He has hypertension" but "He is hypertensioning." While doing a physical examination I would keep talking to the patient while regularly checking his blood pressure. I discovered I could make that pressure go up or down — not by what I was saying or asking, but by what I was making happen in the person's head. Naturally, I found patients with no anger who had high blood pressure and people with horrible jobs and nasty spouses who did not have high blood pressure. But the ones with high blood pressure did have what is called "anxiety." There, with a little conniving, is where I found an answer . . . not the only answer but one that works.

Anxiety is a common term and one of the mainstays of psychiatric theory. It is defined as an emotion. It isn't. It is a compound of two things: an awareness of the existence of ambiguity and a depressive reaction to this awareness. More simply, it means that you don't know what's going to happen, and you are unhappy about this. And this is exactly what I consistently found in people with elevated blood pressure—that they did, indeed, have an incredible intolerance of ambiguity. I have described a person with high blood pressure as a person with his head in a neck brace—so he can't look up—who must walk through a forest on a narrow, winding path, and who knows that up in *one* of those trees there is a very large and very hungry boa constrictor waiting just for him. Do you get the picture?

The awareness of ambiguity is not a bad and unpleasant thing but a *good* thing, a major survival mechanism. It is to be welcomed as a warning sign saying, "Attention! Be careful!" And we learn that with proper attention to this warning, great success will come our way in getting things accomplished.

For example, suppose *you are* driving the freeway. The traffic is heavy and you begin to feel jittery. You don't know what that turkey in the next lane is going to do. You have several choices. You can keep getting more nervous and/or angry. You can get off the freeway and pop a Valium or you can have a cocktail which will seem to resolve your problem but will not improve your chances of reaching your destination. Or you can drive carefully and watch everything around you like a hawk. (There are, of course times when a brief coffee stop or a rest or taking surface streets is a bright idea.)

We have looked carefully at the thinking behind high blood pressure and found that this thought pattern is not unique to the hypertensive person but common to all people. The person with high blood pressure just does it more and better. Further, it means that the common garden variety of hypertension can be prevented — or can be treated while it is still "labile" (when pressure goes up under stress and down when the stress is over). We can continue now and list those things that I advise not only for the person with high blood pressure but for the treatment or prevention of any kind of problem.

• Learn to quickly identify the onset of anger and depressive feelings in yourself.

• Pick something you don't want to have happen to you — a heart attack, an ulcer, the removal of some organ — and when something happens that would normally make you become either angry or unhappy, ask yourself if giving in to these negative feelings is worth the disease price you'll have to pay. If the answer is yes, seek professional help, preferably from a therapist who is *not* depressed.

• Discontinue any medications that are central nervous system depressants — this includes many of the drugs now so frequently prescribed.

• Use alcohol only in *trivial* amounts: It's probably the worst brain depressant we have.

• Start observing other people: their postures, their choice of words and tones of voice, pitch, and stress. Study the reactions of others and try to guess what is going on in their heads. And then watch yourself. A good item to start with is shoulder posture: down and forward is depressed, up and forward is hostile, up and back gives you the feeling that you are working toward the control of your own reality. Try these postures alternately and observe your own reactions and those of others to these postures. You'll be amazed.

• Decide each morning that throughout the day whatever happens will not make you as angry or as unhappy as it would have the day before.

• Get rid of the words "got to," "have to," "should," "must," "ought to," and that old favorite, "willpower." You *can't* do anything except what you want to do — so enjoy it.

There are obviously many more guidelines that I could list and undoubtedly many more I have not seen. But these are, at least, a start in the right direction. Believe it or not, such behaviors help with the "real" medical problems; whether abnormal gastric acidity, elevated cholesterol, or a pimple on your nose is your particular problem.

And for the curious — what were the results of this approach to hypertension in my practice? Previously uncontrolled patients could be brought down to normal levels (below 140/90 mmHg) utilizing only thiazide diuretic medication, and thus avoiding the complex-acting and unpleasant ganglionic blocking agents, many of which, by the way, have depressing effects. Many patients learned that their "early" hypertension could be eradicated. Typical of one of these was a person who for years had been found to have elevated blood pressure upon each consultation with a new doctor. And the blood pressure would fall with rest, reassurance from the new doctor, and the like. These patients, I believe, are the pool from which later fixed hypertensives are developed: other doctors claim that this entity is meaningless and no risk. I do not agree. Finally, as far as results, when I closed my practice I had *no* paralyzed patients lying in nursing homes waiting out the dreary years.

It is my carefully considered opinion that negative states, particularly anger and depression, are critical components in the development of all the most common medical and psychiatric problems we can get — and this includes cancer. And I do believe that by learning how our heads work and how to work our heads, we can all learn to live longer, healthier, and happier lives.

THE HEALING BRAIN

By Douglas Garr

It is another hectic morning in a cramped neurophysiology laboratory. Hunched over his microscope, a researcher focuses on a nerve cell taken from the spinal cord of a mouse. He will hook up an amplifier to measure the neuron's activity, then punch the results into a computer.

Yesterday's figures light up the video display, and Dr. Jeffrey Barker, casually dressed in a blue turtleneck, checks them and nods. Dr. Barker and his assistant break into an arcane language fraught with references to synapses, dendrites, and axons. Brainspeak. If not for the Haydn on the stereo, a couple of stray fish tanks, and his daughter's playful crayon drawings, Barker's lab might belong to the ill-fated Dr. Jekyll.

But Barker's work at the National Institute of Neurological and Communicative Disorders and Stroke, in Bethesda, Maryland, is decidedly beneficial. "We're trying to find out how nerve cells communicate," he says. "We're taking the central nervous system apart. Right now all we have is unidentified flying neurons."

Thirty miles to the northeast, at Johns Hopkins Medical School, in Baltimore, Dr. Caroline Bedell Thomas is doing some very different sleuthing. Dr. Thomas has no fancy scientific hardware. Instead, she relies on questionnaires and the U. S. Postal Service.

In one of the longest-running studies ever conducted, Thomas asked 1,337 Johns Hopkins medical students who graduated between 1948 and 1964 to undergo a battery of psychological and biological tests—while they were students. She's been checking their health ever since. The experiment, known as the Precursors Study, was designed to uncover the medical effects of dozens of mental and physical factors from alcohol consumption and cigarette smoking to anxiety and depression.

As the first students reach middle age—some have already died—Thomas is beginning to draw some preliminary conclusions. Those students whose personalities she calls "irregular-uneven"—brilliant, moody, over- or under-demanding, and over- or undercautious—developed cancer, hypertension, or coronary occlusions much more often than the "slow-solid" or "rapidfacile" types. The "irregular-unevens" are considerably more likely to die younger than the other groups.

Though Barker's and Thomas's studies appear to have little in common, they—and many related projects—are contributing to a fundmental change in clinical medicine. From two distinct vantage points—Barker probing inside and

Thomas peeking in from the outside—they are discovering that the brain exerts far more control over our bodies than we ever imagined possible.

Doctors once saw the brain as little more than a sophisticated computer nearly independent of the body, which carried it almost as a parasite. That view started to change with the "chemical revolution" in the Seventies. First came the discovery that the brain manufactures endorphins and enkephalines, opiatelike substances that relieve pain and stress. More recently researchers have noticed that the brain is responsible for a variety of hormonal and chemical activities that affect our appetite, our blood pressure, and even our sex drive.

"It is quite clear that the brain is connected to everything else in a way that's beyond our understanding," says Dr. Robert Orenstein, of the Institute for the Study of Human Knowledge. "We've had to step back enormously in awe, as ordinary people, and in less awe, as scientists."

We've known for some time that anxiety and depression can worsen such illnesses as diabetes, asthma, headaches, peptic ulcers, and cardiovascular disorders. For more than two decades Dr. Hans Selye, a Nobel laureate and founder of the International Institute for Stress, in Montreal, has been publicizing the psychic battleground and its physical implications.

The author of 38 books on stress and health, Dr. Selye believes that peaceful thoughts release beneficial hormones while fearful ones let out harmful hormones. Cortisone, in Selye's words, is "a tissue tranquilizer," and adrenalin causes us to be aggressive. But Selye is careful to note that stress is a normal part of life. "You can't make many generalizations, because some people take stress very well and others don't," he says.

René Dubos, the Pulitzer Prize-winning author and reowned microbiologist at Rockefeller University, offers a case in point. Now eighty, Dr. Dubos recalls his first wife's death nearly four decades ago with startling clarity. In 1942 she contracted tuberculosis, and Dubos says he was able to trace the origins of her illness to her childhood. Her father was a painter of china, and she was exposed to silica, a compound that might have promoted the development of TB. With standard medical treatment, she was partially cured and led a fairly normal life.

After two years, however, the disease reappeared. Dubos remembers attending a concert at New York's Carnegie Hall some time later. While walking along Fifty-seventh Street, his wife, a former pianist, became sullen when she realized she could no longer play. "Two weeks later she was dead," Dubos says. Though he doesn't claim that she died because she was upset, he realized that her depression might have exacerbated her illness. "The evidence of the psychological component in disease is overwhelming," Dubos now concludes.

Backed by a torrent of scientific papers, such incidents have caught the attention of doctors across the country. When author Norman Cousins contracted a rare and painful connective-tissue disease, physicians gave him a 1-in-500 chance of recovering fully. But Cousins took an active, aggressive role in his fight, often ignoring the dictates of conventional medicine. He left the hospital earlier than he was supposed to, took charge of his own therapy, and watched Marx Brothers movies, hoping that humor would ease his pain. After he recovered, Cousins wondered, "Does this mean that laughter stimulated production of the endorphins?"

Science hasn't yet answered his question. The same question has occurred to many physicians. When Cousins wrote about his illness in the *New England Journal of Medicine,* 3,000 doctors responded with letters.

Stress effects can be subtle, according to Dr. Barney Dlin, a psychiatrist at Temple University, in Philadelphia, who has found a correlation between emotion and coronary disease. "For example, in our study we worked with a patient who had a heart attack when his child was four years old. We learned in our interview that his father had suffered a heart attack when the patient was four years old," Dr. Dlin noted in the journal *Psychosomatics*. "Consciously or unconsciously, a patient may forecast his own sickness or death."

And at the University of Maryland Medical School, psychologist James Lynch has conducted numerous clinical studies of emotion and its relation to blood pressure and heart disease. Though he commands a laboratory full of impressive monitoring equipment, Dr. Lynch is often more fascinated by the intangible factors that influence human health.

He likes to point to a 1965 study of heart disease in the United States: Nevada had one of the highest rates; neighboring Utah, the lowest. What caused such a disparity? Obviously, it wasn't a simple answer like the quality of water or air or the medium-income level. There were nearly identical in the two states. But the people of Utah generally are very religious; the state has a stable population and an unusually low divorce rate. Nevada's principal industry is gambling. The state's inhabitants are often transient, and Nevada's divorce rate is triple Utah's.

Perhaps the explanation lay somewhere in the patient's mind, Lynch speculated. Could it be that loneliness had something to do with heart disease? In those days that was a brash proposal.

Lynch found the mortality statistics for heart disease in the United States are two to five times higher among unmarried people than among married. Obviously, Lynch admits, being single doesn't mean you're automatically destined to suffer a heart attack. But he thinks it would pay medical science to study the problem further. Lynch isn't optimistic that the research will take place, however. "Can you imagine writing a grant proposal for a project on love?" he asks rhetorically.

How is it that the brain affects our ability to resist illness? One likely route is through the immune system. In one study, the hypothalamus, a section of the brain that regulates the pituitary hormones, has been linked with the body's ability to form antibodies to fight off infection. And recent research on one kind of infection-fighting white blood cell, the T lymphocyte, reveals the presence of brain hormones on the cell's outer membrane.

It is far from certain just how important this link between the brain and the immune system will prove. But scientists have speculated that a few of our healthy cells may turn malignant each day. The white blood cells, they suspect, recognize this transformation and destroy the cells before the cancer spreads. So if someone does contract an infection or develop cancer, his body's immune system may have broken down. Then the connection could be very important indeed.

One of the more striking examples occurred two years ago in Fort Lupton, Colorado. Jim Kunzman, a farmer, suddenly had to contend with the loss of his two young children, who were killed in an automobile accident. Kunzman, whose story was documented on film, found that he had lost interest in his work and in his life. Though never sick in the past, he began to feel ill, slept long hours, and lost his appetite. Eighteen months after his children had died, doctors found he had multiple myeloma, a bone cancer. Kunzman underwent chemotherapy, but its side effects only made him feel worse. Then, early in 1980, he began seeing a psychologist and taking about his feelings. Remarkably his cancer regressed. Today he's actively tilling his farmland.

"My immune system was at a very low ebb," Kunzman now says evenly. "I think that subconsciously I wanted to punish myself in some way, and my body simply obliged me."

Oncologists are very careful to note that Kunzman's cancer might have disappeared for any number of reasons. But no one discounts the possibility that his sickness and subsequent good health had a psychological basis.

In fact, physicians at the Cancer Counseling Research Center, in Fort Worth, Texas, have turned this idea into a practical — and highly successful — cancer treatment. Developed by Stephanie Matthews-Simonton, a psychologist, and Dr. Carl Simonton, a radiation oncologist, the center's treatment program focuses on the psychology factor in cancer. The Simontons combine conventional psychotherapy with such standard medical techniques as radiation and chemotherapy.

Though the Simontons are careful not to make any miracle claims for their success stories, the results have been encouraging. In the past five years their 200 patients have survived an average of twice as long as cancer victims who received only medical treatment. Some of the patients at the research center have had their cancer disappear completely.

The Simontons' technique grew out of experiments with biofeedback, which enjoyed its greatest popularity in the late Sixties and early Seventies. During the biofeedback studies, Mrs. Simonton says, she and her husband began to ask themselves, "If a person could be taught to influence heart rate, blood flow, and blood pressure, all physiological systems under the autonomic nervous system, could people be taught to put energy into building their immune system?"

The first patient they experimented on was a sixty-one-year-old man with advanced, probably fatal, throat cancer. (The Simontons publish scientific papers only on patients who are diagnosed as having 12 to 18 months to live.) In addition to radiation treatment, the Simontons asked the man to relax and visualize a pleasant setting for a few minutes, three times a day: a quiet mountain scene or an idyllic setting by a stream. Later the patient began to visualize his tumor. Then he was told to think about his body's white blood cells invading the tumor in his throat and eventually destroying it.

In two months his throat cancer went into remission. "What was astonishing," Mrs. Simonton says, "was not so much that his tumor shrank—which you would expect during radiation treatment—but that he experienced nothing in the way of side effects." The man got stronger, gained weight, and became cheerful. "When arthritis began to bother him, he turned his white blood cells on that, and it cleared up," she adds.

Soon the Simontons began to notice distinct emotional similarities among their cancer patients. "Typically what we saw was a high-stress pattern six to eighteen months before the diagnosis of cancer," Mrs. Simonton reports. "Frequently there will be a real or imagined loss of some kind—death of a spouse, a child leaving home—leading to a profound despair. This is something that the cancer-prone personality has a lot of difficulty dealing with, the mind-body connection."

The idea that cancer patients share a broad psychological profile is new and controversial. There are, after all, thousands of carcinogens to which many of us are exposed every day; any of them can surely cause death after 15 or 20 years of exposure.

In the late Fifties Lawrence LeShan, a clinical psychologist who practices on Manhattan's Upper West Side, developed the notion that people who got cancer had certain psychological traits in common. This idea was scoffed at. Today LeShan smiles wryly when he recalls the resistance that greeted his wish to conduct a study to confirm his idea. Thinking he was a charlatan, the administrators of hospitals and cancer clinics refused to let him interview terminal patients.

Finally, though, LeShan was allowed to talk with cancer patients at a program run by the Institute for Applied Biology. Two patterns began to emerge. First, he found cancer patients lacked a strong will to live. Second, the patients found it difficult to express their anger or resentment.

In one experiment, considering psychological factors alone, LeShan was able to predict correctly who had cancer in 24 of 28 cases. Of 22 "terminal" cancer patients whom he began treating a decade ago, 12 are still alive.

Since then, two Rochester, New York doctors have tried to guess—again basing their guess on personality traits—which of the women who entered the hospital for cervical biopsies actually had cancer. They were right 72 percent of the time.

Though we have grown to accept the theory of the cancer-prone personality, LeShan hints that American clinics may be lagging behind those in the rest of the world. During a trip abroad he was startled to find great interest in the psychological treatment of cancer. "In West Germany," he learned, "if you want to set up a cancer clinic, you can't get federal funding unless you agree to set up a psychological rehabilitation ward."

All this raises some questions: How do the patients who survive cancer react to their illness? Do they take an active role, as author Norman Cousins did? Or do they remain passive?

"What we're seeing," Mrs. Simonton finds, "is that the ornery, scrappy, cantankerous patient does better than the passive, compliant, sweet, denying patient who bottles everything up inside."

LeShan adds, "Bad patients do better than good patients. The oncologists know this, but they haven't really come to grips with it."

One of the mind's most puzzling influences on the body appears in cases of chronic pain. Pain is subjective; it is the brain that feels it and decides how severe it is. We've known for years that soldiers wounded in battle often don't feel pain until hours later. And in dozens of studies doctors have reported that ordinary sugar pills or salt pills relieve pain in up to half of the patients who take them. Recently researchers have suggested that the placebo, though it has no direct effect, eases pain by triggering the release of enkephalins in the brain. Anthropologists have even seen primitive cultures in which the husband feels pains during his wife's labor and the woman seems comfortable.

It seems that our culture has a great influence on how we feel pain. Dr. Richard Black, codirector of the Pain Treatment Center at Johns Hopkins, believes that he has seen the proof among his own patients. "We have found some interesting sociological problems with our own chronic-pain patients," he says. "Some have what I guardedly call inadequate personalities. They have never been able to hold down a job; when they do, they get injured frequently. They're always running for the pill or the bottle. A high percentage tend to be child abusers and were abused as children themselves. So you are dealing with a deep-seated problem that goes on from generation to generation."

Dr. Black says that pain patients are often misdiagnosed, frequently because of psychology. He recalls the case of one patient, a fifty-two year old woman who'd had a mastectomy seven years earlier. She was technically cured, and although her arm was swollen and her chest was scarred, she experienced only mild pain.

"Then her next-door neighbor got a fulminating carcinoma of the breast and died within six months," Black reports. "This was a neighbor our patient hardly knew, but she had an intense grief reaction nevertheless." Soon afterward the woman sought out another doctor and complained to him of severe pain.

"He diagnosed her as hurting rather than having an anxiety attack," Black continues. "He gave her a painkiller and a tranquilizer to help her sleep. Both drugs, because of their chemical effect on the central nervous system, made the woman feel depressed. When you're depressed, everything's worse and you hurt more. Meanwhile the doctor had done nothing to ease her anxiety. In fact, by doing nothing, he had made it worse."

One of Black's colleagues at Johns Hopkins, Dr. Nelson Hendler, saw so many patients with back pain that he devised a ten-minute psychological test to sift out people who lack an apparent "organic" basis for their pain. Dr. Hendler says the "objective" pain patient has "a history of stability, a sense of independence, and a resentment of incapacitation."

Hendler is also director of the Mensana Clinic, a pain center in Stevenson, Maryland. At Mensana, treatment concentrates on the behavioral aspects of pain. The patients take responsibility for their own medication. There are no nurses to coddle them. "In group therapy, patients are encouraged to talk about their pain, sort of like Pain Anonymous," Hendler says.

As clinical medicine is adjusting to our new understanding of the brain's role in health, neuroscience is ferreting out still newer insights. For example, Dr. Quentin Pittman, assistant professor of pharmacology at the University of Calgary, in Alberta, Canada, and his colleague, Dr. Warren Veale, have discovered that the brain may control fever. During the experiments, Drs. Pittman and Veale noticed that newborn lambs never developed a fever; so the pharmacologists began to search for natural substances that might repress fever.

What they found was vasopressin, a hormone first discovered in the Fifties. Acting on the kidneys, vasopressin controls the body's water content and helps regulate blood pressure. And, according to Pittman and Veale, the higher the level of vasopressin in a test subject's bloodstream, the lower the fever.

"As a result, we have come to suspect that the brain has its own type of aspirin," Pittman says, much as it has its own morphinelike substances. "The next question is obvious: Is there some way we can stimulate the body to produce its own aspirin?" If so, he hopes, we may soon be able to eliminate a headache at will.

And brain research is just beginning to help us understand our sex drive. In 1971 scientists first isolated a substance known as LH-RH (for luteinizing hormone-releasing hormone) in the pituitary gland. Shortly thereafter Dr. Robert Moss, of the Dallas-Southwestern Medical School's department of physiology, found that LH-RH induced sexual activity in female rats, even after the animals' adrenal and pituitary glands had been removed. "The only place LH-RH could have acted was in the brain," Dr. Moss concluded.

Moss repeated the tests on other animals, both male and female, with similar results. In humans, however, LH-RH seldom worked, except when it was given to people with sexual dysfuncions. "Still," Moss reflects, "the idea of chemical reactions affecting neural activity . . . we've just scratched the surface."

The work continues. Dr. Barker, in Bethesda, is struggling to find out how brain cells talk to one another. Someday he may identify some of his flying neurons. Dr. Thomas, at Johns

Hopkins, continues to collect data on her surviving medical students, helping to unravel the physical and psychological bases of cancer, heart disease, and even suicide. She has published 80 papers so far, and another researcher will probably pick up where she leaves off.

Scientists are beginning to look at memory as a physiological problem. Is senility simply an inevitable part of old age, or is it an ailment that can be evaded or cured? Dr. Dubos likens the brain to a muscle. If not exercised, it atrophies in every way.

At the neurological-research arm of the National Institutes of Health, there is already talk of neural prostheses for paralyzed limbs: Why can't a microcomputer, activated by brain waves and embedded in that limb, be programmed to control basic motor functions? It may soon happen.

Meanwhile the mold of Western medicine is slowly wearing away and being recut. "I've seen a swami take random spots on his hand and raise the temperature on one and lower it on the other." LeShan marvels. "But what does this do? We can get an alpha wave and control our electroencephalogram, but why? What's the value?

"Everyone expects the easy route to health, but it cannot be done in two weekends. People think that if they jog and if they take ten extra milligrams of vitamin C a day, zinc, and so on, they'll be sexually attractive and will live forever. But it doesn't work that way."

How it does work, we're not exactly sure. Today's studies of the brain will eventually show us the path.

THE NEW BIOFEEDBACK

By Bob Kall

Biofeedback, the hip fad that promised cosmic consciousness and panacean answers to human ills, is dead. But rising from its ashes is a new, practical biofeedback, an electron microscope of inner space, that has been validated by thousands of published research studies. NASA astronauts already use it to overcome zero-gravity motion sickness. Stroke patients use it to reactivate paralyzed limbs by mentally activating muscles, one nerve cell at a time. It helps epileptics abort their seizures and headache sufferers ease their pain without drugs. Athletes fine-tune their movements to the new biofeedback, and people learn to hear sounds beyond their normal hearing range.

Feedback can be applied to almost any measurable behavior. It's an added tool that allows more information to flow between the mind and the body. Biofeedback simultaneously isolates, magnifies, and feeds back information about tiny, normally imperceptible behavior changes as they occur. This amplified information helps the individual to influence those inner changes.

Practical biofeedback requires the combined application of effective hardware and a subject willing to practice long and hard on the machine. It is no miracle, not even a mystery. In the past, biofeedback was seen as impractical because the required equipment was expensive and laboratory-bound. But technological advances have reduced size and cost to the point where the techniques are beginning to have importance in real life.

A good example of this is NASA researcher Pat Cowling's pill-sized, swallowable stomach-activity monitor. It emits a radio signal so she can check gastrointestinal reactions to "zero-gravity sickness syndrome," which, she says, is the space program's highest-priority biomedical-research problem. Working with such devices, researchers at the Ames Research Center, in California, have developed a training program centered on a highly choreographed BF course that teaches space travelers how to minimize the physical effects of zero gravity.

Subjects are taught to control their heart and breathing rates, blood flow to the face and hands, the activity of key muscles, and electrical conductivity of their skin. Then they have to perform a coordinated pattern of these maneuvers while sitting in a centrifugal chair that spins faster and faster, subjecting them to greater stresses.

Cowling says modestly that it looks as if biofeedback is getting better results than such alternatives as drugs and attempts to simulate the effects of movement under zero gravity. The drugs have negative side effects, and simulations such as spinning the astronauts in centrifugal chairs are slower and do not seem to transfer to real zero-g conditions.

Soon she plans to try BF training to lower astronauts' oxygen requirements and control their core body temperatures during emergencies.

Back on Earth, Keith Sedlacek, M.D., director of New York's Stress Regulation Institute, predicts that with employee health-care costs going sky high, BF will soon be adopted for on-the-job stress control. "It's cost-effective preventive medicine. Executives will get BF access included with their key to the executive washroom. Blue-collar workers and middle-management executives will get group training. You'll wear telemetry equipment while you work so that high-stress activities encountered on the job can be detected and dealt with," Sedlacek says. He has already begun training executives to reduce high blood pressure and reduce stress.

Tom Budzynski, clinical director of the Biofeedback Institute, of Denver, who never read Larry Niven's description of fictional "autodocs," gives a pretty close description of what real ones might be like. "You'd wake up in the morning and plug yourself in to a device that would tell you what in your body would need to be adjusted to maintain optimal health. You could wear the device like a wristwatch. It would sound warnings whenever a physiological system went out of a preset normal range. Using teleme-try, the monitor would produce computer-gener-ated video displays on your TV, showing you what's wrong by using programs from linked cen-tral-storage libraries."

If you work in a job where you stay in the same position all day, feedback equipment may help re-lieve strain. You'll attach a joint angle monitor to your hip or knee, a pressure transducer on your chair, or a strain gauge on your back. When you're in the right position, they will remain si-lent. But you'll get a warning if you move too far from the healthiest, most efficient posture. The feedback will cut your risk of back pain and muscle aches and will bring you more energy on the job.

John Basmajian, M.D., a world-renowned re-habilitation expert, applies another BF technique to revive the muscles of paralyzed stroke patients. These people have to learn how to use their mus-cles all over again. Muscles are composed of groups of motor units, each controlled by a single cell in the spinal cord. Dr. Basmajian uses needle-thin microelectrodes to feed back the activity of a single motor group. Each nerve impulse causes a sound. That way, even the smallest amount of surviving muscle control can be measured through repetition.

After just a few days or weeks of practice, some of the patients were able to send Morse code BF signals by controlling their single-celled motor neurons. Basmajian says, "People have much better inherent ability to control internal behavior if they are given biofeedback. Training for improved muscle performance is one of bio-feedback's most proven uses."

Other researchers have been training people to activate parts of the brain and turn on different brain-wave frequencies. Epileptics are being taught to abort seizures by producing a preventive brainwave pattern. Psychiatric patients listen better when they produce brain waves that make them more receptive to suggestion. Bright, intuitively street-wise ghetto children are right-brain dominant; but they can improve their reading and mathematical abilities, which require analytical, logical thinking, by using biofeedback to increase the activity of their left brain hemisphere.

Already computers have been connected with electroencephalographic (EEG) brain-wave monitors. They turn tape recordings or video terminals on and off, depending on an individual's brain-wave state. This technology is still in its infancy, but eventually you'll be able to enhance your reading speed and information retention by working with a video screen connected to an EEG monitor. The rate the words are presented will be determined by your brain-wave activity. The color of the screen, the size of the letters, the audio background all will be modulated to maximize your brain's receptivity.

With simpler technology, hyperactive children are already watching TV and slide shows this way. The program is turned on only when the kids relax their muscles enough.

After muscle biofeedback, thermal feedback training to increase blood flow is probably the most common BF technique used today. Blood, heated at the body's core, distributes warmth to the skin and limbs. Peripheral-blood-flow regulation is one of the most easily mastered self-control techniques. It's used to relieve migraine headaches, chronic pain, arthritis, menstrual discomfort, high blood pressure, skin diseases, and stress disorders. Even Raynaud's syndrome, a disease in which hands, usually responding to cold weather or air conditioning, get painfully cold because of decreased blood circulation, has been alleviated with BF. It's even been shown to speed the healing of burns.

For all its benefits, we still don't understand how BF works. Ed Taub, president of the Biofeedback Society of America, doesn't see this as a problem. The actions of drugs, he argues, are also poorly understood. We test them to make sure they're safe and to see what they do: then we use them, even if the mechanism for their operation isn't fully understood. BF, he believes, is at the same stage, and will remain so until much more is learned about the brain and its supporting network of nerves.

SUDDEN DEATH

By Patrick Huyghe

One third of all the people who die a natural
death in the United States do so by taking that
quick, frightful leap into oblivion known as sudden death. Doctors define this as rapid, unexpected death occurring in seemingly healthy
people. Most of these fatalities are the result of
heart failure, and normally some heart disease
can be found to explain them. But since many
people with severe cardiovascular deterioration
live long and useful lives, doctors have begun to
wonder whether other contributing factors are
involved. They also wonder whether these same
factors might not be behind the 25,000 or so
deaths each year that are not only sudden but unexplained as well.

Leading the list of causes is something that has
been the focus of much medical research in recent
years: an intense emotion. The idea that emotions can provoke sudden death has had wide-

spread acceptance ever since civilization began. History and folklore are full of stories about people dying in the throes of some powerful emotion. History tells us, for example, that one Chilon of Lacedaemon made his exit because of an overdose of joy while embracing his son, who had just carried away a prize at the Olympic Games. Almost 2,000 years ago the Roman scholar of medicine Celsus wrote that emotional states could affect the heart — an opinion that William Harvey, the seventeenth-century physician and discoverer of the human circulatory system, shared.

The idea fell into disrepute in the late nineteenth century once the fledgling science of modern medicine declared all causes of death could be determined at the autopsy table, but now those venerable observations are being reexamined, and there is a solid body of evidence linking emotions to destabilized heartbeats and, ultimately, to death.

With improved medical services and the advent of techniques like cardiopulmonary resuscitation, many people now survive serious heart attacks, and this fact has allowed some researchers to talk to the victims and find out what their emotional states were just before the attack. Doctors at Boston's Brigham and Women's Hospital did this very thing last year with one group of heart-attack victims. They found that, of 117 resuscitated patients, about a fifth reported some acute emotional disturbance just before their near-fatal arrhythmias, seriously abnormal heartbeats that can culminate in death. Among the disturbances they listed: bitter arguments, some public humiliation, marital problems, business failures, profound grief, and, in one case, nightmares.

"There is strong evidence for a link between stress and sudden cardiac death," says Dr. Regis DeSilva, a cardiologist involved in the study, "but the association still lacks definitive scientific proof." The chief problem, he says is that it is hard to translate emotions like despair and fear into something that can be measured. What evidence there is does suggest that things like stress, fear, hopelessness, and even the act of heavy breathing can activate the sympathetic nervous system, the part that marshals energy for instant use, the "fight or flight" response. Switching on this nervous system, doctors say, can trigger arrhythmias and cardiac arrest.

In the 1930s one celebrated doctor in India demonstrated the power of the mind and imagination in an astonishing and deadly experiment he performed on a criminal who had been condemned to death. The doctor wanted to learn whether the human imagination could kill. The convict was an assassin of distinguished rank, and court permission had been obtained to bleed him to death inside prison so that his family might be spared the disgrace of a public hanging. When the time came, the condemned man was blindfolded, led into a room, and strapped to a table. Under it a container was set up to drip water gently into a basin on the floor. The doctor pricked the skin of the man's arms and legs near his veins as if to bleed him and at the same time started the water dripping. The convict believed that the dripping he heard was his blood flowing out, and when the sound of the dripping water at length stopped, he passed out and died — without actually losing one drop of blood.

Of all psychological stresses, it appears that fright is the one most likely to cause rapid and sudden death. George Engel, a psychiatrist at the University of Rochester School of Medicine, in New York, has collected 170 case histories of emotional sudden death and found that more than a quarter of them involve some "setting of personal danger or threat of injury, real or symbolic." The list includes cases of terrified patients who died just before a minor surgical procedure. For this reason some surgeons refuse to operate on patients who fear surgery.

If there is any light at the end of this dark tunnel, it may come from one unusual group of victims whose deaths may offer some clues to exactly how these sudden cardiac deaths occur. These are the Asian refugees in this country who have been particularly susceptible to so-called nightmare deaths. They constitute the single largest category of unexplained sudden deaths yet discovered.

In the past four years about 40 Laotians, Vietnamese, and Kampucheans have died mysteriously in their sleep. The victims were mostly young, apparently healthy, men. Death in each instance happened at night and took only a matter of minutes. This strange pattern had first been noted in the 1940s and 1950s among young men in Japan, where the disease is called *pokkuri,* and among Filipino men in the Philippines and Hawaii, where it is known as *bangungut* (the Tagalog word for "nightmare"). Autopsies done on the men revealed they had suffered acute cardiac failure, but none had underlying heart disease. And because some deaths were preceded by heavy breathing, groaning, and screaming, there was a popular notion the deaths were caused by nightmares.

If doctors can find out exactly what happened among these refugees, says Dr. Roy Baron, an epidemiologist at the Center for Disease Control who is in charge of the investigation of such cases, they may well have a clue as to what caused other inexplicable sudden deaths. Cardiac pathologists who studied heart tissue taken from people recently deceased think the heart failure may have originated from some abnormality in the heart's connective tissue, its electrical system. Perhaps the best way to locate the triggering factor involved, Baron suggests, is to find people who have survived these episodes and then study them in sleep laboratories.

"I don't think we are going to get very far by arguing these people had a bad dream and scared themselves to death," adds Dr. Merrill Mitler, a sleep physiologist and chief of the sleep Disorders Center at the State University of New York at Stony Brook. Right now the leading hypothesis which is not inconsistent with the autopsy and case history material collected by Dr. Baron, Mitler says, is that REM (rapid-eye-movement) sleep precipitates a kind of cardiovascular crisis.

The respiratory pattern becomes highly irregular during REM. For vulnerable individuals, sleep can be fraught with risks. At times it can seriously alter the pulse rate. Partly for these reasons, most nocturnal heart attacks occur during REM.

"While everyone shows some cardiac irregularity during REM sleep," Mitler asserts, "there may be a subgroup who exhibit terrific cardiac irregularities during REM. What we would like to do is study that subgroup in which these night deaths are most frequent and see whether we can find any exaggeration of normal cardiac and respiratory irregularities."

Studies like Mitler's may eventually help pinpoint some of the high-risk factors. Meanwhile the mystery of sudden death remains an awesome one.

BEYOND THE BRAIN

By Sir John Eccles

Every day of our lives we face a strange paradox. While we take it for granted our minds act on our brains—that is, by merely thinking a thought, we can direct our brains to make any movement we wish—most philosophers, psychologists, and neuroscientists say this commonsense belief is wrong. They assert, dogmatically, that because mental events like thought and planning an action are not of the material world, they cannot cause changes anywhere in that world, not even in the brain.

Those who make these statements believe that all our actions are entirely dependent on the brain, even though we have the feeling that it is thought or desire that controls our voluntary movements. What these materialists allege is that the neural events involved in any voluntary movement give us this false impression. The explanation for this is something they label an identity relationship. There is an outward movement we can see, and there is a mental event associated with it. It is not a case of one causing the other, but rather they are the same event looked at from different perspectives, inside and outside. As a result, whenever the nerve cells are firing, we perceive that we are causing it, but in fact it is merely an illusion.

These same theorists go on to claim that eventually neuroscientists will be able to identify, in more and more detail, the neural events behind the whole range of conscious experiences — the excitement of creativity, joy, even love. Eventually, they say, everything will be explained by nerve-cell activities, if not in our lifetime, in the lifetimes of generations to come. For that reason the philosopher Sir Karl Popper derisively labels this reductionist program promissory materialism, since it essentially "promises" to explain everything someday.

But don't be alarmed. I believe we should not take these dogmatic statements too seriously, because they are based on prejudice and on knowledge that is most inadequate. The reality of the action of the mind is cruelly brought home to anyone afflicted with a disease such as Parkinsonism, a nervous disease in which the person afflicted suffers from involuntary muscle tremors and a general slowing down and weakening of bodily movement. Here there is no identity relationship. Diseased individuals find great difficulty in carrying out a planned action, no matter how much they desire it. If they were so afflicted, those philosophers who speak so glibly about the simplicity of the mind/body problem would soon realize that there is an immensely complex neural machinery of the brain interposed between the intention to act and the action itself.

Let me illustrate what is involved in some planned action such as lifting a glass of wine elegantly to one's lips, or making a skillful golf stroke. Simple though these motions seem, they are the outcome of events in the body's nervous system that, at a conservative estimate, involve hundreds of millions of neurons. Think of all the muscles that have to be made to contract with just the right strength and timing. A golf stroke, for example, brings into play almost all the muscles of the limbs, torso, neck, and head. Years of training are necessary to learn these skills. Although an expert player may have little knowledge of how his individual muscles are performing, he knows by how he moves and how precisely he hits the ball whether his neural machinery is operating smoothly or not.

We know something of the intricacies of muscle action from scientific studies of champion shot-putters and of gymnasts performing simple exercises, but we can only imagine the subtleties of the interrelated muscle contractions that occur in the highly skilled performances of musicians, dancers, actors, athletes, and technicians manipulating delicate instruments. For each of us, life is one long symphony of movements that we have been learning since childhood and that are as unique to each of us as the writing of our signature.

I have criticized many times the theories of the

promissory materialists. What I see as an alternate hypothesis is a common-sense belief originally formulated by René Descartes in the seventeenth century and updated by Karl Popper and me. It is called dualist interactionism. It holds that we live in two distinct worlds, the world of the mind and the material world, which includes the brain (the dualism), and that there is an intense interaction across this frontier between the mind and the brain (hence the interactionism).

Until recently this idea had to be assimilated with evidence that the action of the mind was diffused throughout the brain, a "ghost in the machine," but in the last four years this concept has been transformed by three scientific investigations that have identified a special area of the cerebral cortex where mental events cause neural events. It was first discovered in 1943 by neurosurgeon Dr. Wilder Penfield, who named it the supplementary motor area (SMA). The SMA lies on the upper midsurface of each cerebral hemisphere immediately underneath the skull. Ever since its discovery, the SMA has had a disappointing press concerning its role in carrying out bodily movement. The reason for this was that its influences were so imprecise when compared with the brain's true motor cortex, where the areas that control specific parts of the body can be laid out on a quite precise strip map of the brain. But now, in a Cinderella-like transformation, the SMA seems destined to be cast in the role of master control of all voluntary movement.

The most remarkable studies illustrating this

have been done by neurologist Dr. Nils Lassen and his colleagues at the Neurological Institute in Copenhagen. They have built a wonderful machine that measures changes in the circulation of the blood through small regions of the cerebral cortex, and by so doing, they can measure the intensity of nerve-cell activities within it. To do this, they first inject a small amount of a radioactive tracer, 133 xenon, in solution into a patient's internal carotid artery, which carries blood to the brain. (It should be mentioned here that a tube had already been inserted to make an angiogram, an X ray of the blood vessels, for therapeutic purposes and that the patients willingly gave a few minutes of their time for the innocuous injection procedure.) Radiation from the injected cerebral hemisphere is recorded by 254 Geiger counters arranged in a helmet that the patient wears. During the injection the patient performs a learned repetitive task for 60 seconds. At the same time the radioactive pattern of the underlying brain activity is computed for each of the 254 sites and then played out as 15-color mosaic map of the brain, showing any changes in brain activity.

The patient is asked to do a series of finger-thumb movements that requires total concentration. He has to touch his thumb to each finger in turn following a distinct pattern: two touches to the first finger, one to the second, three to the third, two to the fourth. And then he reverses the pattern: two the fourth, three to the third, one to the second, two to the first, and so on back around again until the 60 seconds are up. Anyone who tries this will find that it is impossible to talk or even think of anything else at the same time because it requires so much concentration to get it right.

As expected, Lassen and his group have found a large increase in activity in the area of the motor cortex that controls thumb and finger movements, but there was also a large increase over the SMA. In itself this is an inconclusive result. The SMA, for example, could have been activated after the motor cortex and not before. This possibility was eliminated by a beautiful change in strategy.

The patient was asked to think of the thumb-finger movements in the correct sequence without carrying them out. There is no increased neural activity in the motor cortex, but amazingly the SMA shows almost as large an increase in activity as when the movements are being performed. These results show that, even when a person is only intending to carry out some voluntary act, his thoughts will activate neural events in the SMA and nowhere else.

This conclusion has been corroborated in experiments done by Australian neurophysiologist Dr. Robert Porter, who took recordings of the neurons of a monkey's SMA as the animal voluntarily pulled a lever to get a food reward. Porter found that probably more than a tenth of a second before the motor cortex neurons fired, the SMA cells were activated.

Two German neurologists, Drs. Hans Kornhuber and Luder Deecke, have confirmed this firing order with electrical signals taken from the scalps of people performing voluntary movements. The first electrical sign of nervous activity, called the readiness potential, appears in the scalp region over the SMA, and it is the largest over the SMA throughout the time period — almost a second — before the movement begins.

Most important, they have found that this readiness potential is still large in the SMA of patients afflicted with the severe akinesia, or weakness of movements, of bilateral Parkinsonism, despite the extreme feebleness of the motor act and of the readiness potential over the motor cortex. Again the mental activation of the SMA was found to precede the activity of the motor cortex, which was greatly reduced because of the severe damage to the neural pathway connecting the SMA and the motor cortex.

These experiments have shown that the mind does act on the brain and does it at a precise site in the cerebral cortex. This is only the beginning of our understanding, however. Stretching before us is an immense vista of scientific investigations that have to be done before we can give an account, even in principle, of how we perform any skilled movement. We need to understand how a thought instructs, probably in some coded manner, the neural machinery of the SMA so that the desired voluntary movement results. Also, it is assumed that in the SMA there is an inventory of all learned motor programs, as they are called, and their addresses by which they can be called forth.

Although we still have only a dim understanding of the mystery behind how a person makes any skillful move, what we know already makes the actions of the most sophisticated robot look like a failure by many orders of magnitude when compared to those of a human. It is an exciting and wonderful realization.

Physiologist Sir John Eccles was awarded the 1963 Nobel Prize in Medicine and Physiology for explaining how nerve impulses are transmitted from neuron to neuron.

PART SIX:
OF SCIENCE BORN

CHILDBIRTH 2000

By Gena Corea

Nativity, A.D. 2000. Susan Rogers wants to give birth the old-fashioned way — vaginally. Since most hospital births are done by cesarean section, Susan decides, after her gynecologist confirms her pregnancy, to deliver at home. The midwife — midwives are illegal but omnipresent in America — screens her for risk factors. She finds none.

Toward the end of the pregnancy, while Susan and her husband are relaxing at their home in the woods of Brattleboro, Vermont, a helicopter swoops down and lands in the backyard. A physician and a policeman emerge from the machine and produce a court order authorizing them to take the unborn baby into protective custody to prevent child abuse. They force the screaming woman into the helicopter.

At the hospital, Susan is taken into a birthing suite decorated with houseplants, flowered drapes, and a bedspread. She sits in a rocking chair, stunned, unaware that during her one and only visit to the gynecologist, he registered Susan's pregnancy with the Regional Perinatal Center and implanted in her vagina a tiny receiver for the electronic fetal monitor along with a device used to track down migratory animals.

In the computer room, which looks much like a NASA communications center, obstetricians have been following her pregnancy for months. (Doctors at the center often joke that they are conquering inner space.)

Susan's labor is induced with Pitocin, a stimulant. Two hours later in the computer center behind the suite, the screen displaying her monitoring signal reveals "fetal distress."

The alarm sounds. Susan is rushed into the operating room, strapped to the table, anesthetized. A doctor takes a knife, cuts her abdomen open, and pulls the baby from her womb. Attendants transport the baby to the intensive-care unit for treatment of respiratory distress.

The patient, still dazed, is wheeled back to the homey birthing suite.

This is Norma Swenson's grim vision of childbirth in the year 2000. Swenson, who holds a master's degree from Harvard School of Public Health, is coauthor of *Our Bodies, Ourselves.* Having been active in childbirth groups for twenty years, she is former president of the International Childbirth Education Association (ICEA).

Why do visions of helicopters dance in her head at night? Because this is happening during the day:

• The executive director of the American College of Obstetricians and Gynecologists (ACOG) declared in 1977 that home birth, a growing trend, constituted "child abuse" and "maternal trauma."

• Three home-birth couples—in Louisiana, Idaho, and North Carolina—were accused of child abuse in early 1978. In the North Carolina case, police, acting on an obstetrician's complaint, forcibly took the woman from her home while she was in labor and transported her to a hospital.

• A low-income woman who wanted natural childbirth refused various interventions, including Pitocin injections to speed up her labor, at Boston City Hospital in June 1978. The hospital tried to get a court order forcing her to accept the drug. Then, as her lawyer explained, "There was some concern that this lady must be crazy because she refuses to do what the hospital staff tells her to do." They called in a psychiatrist to judge her mental health while she was in labor. After many hours, they "persuaded" her to accept Pitocin and anesthesia. Several days later, the hospital announced it was instituting proceedings to take her baby on the ground that she might endanger the child. The baby, placed in a foster home for months, has finally been returned to her.

• Dr. Jack M. Schneider, codirector of the Wisconsin Perinatal Center in Madison, has proposed a national registration of pregnancies.

• A "regionalized system of obstetrical treatment," which involves shutting down maternity services in small community hospitals and transporting mothers and infants to large, technologically oriented hospitals, is being established throughout the United States.

Suzanne Arms, author of *Immaculate Deception,* believes that when America has been fully converted to a regionalized obstetrical system, physicians and health authorities will be closely coordinated enough to make Norma Swenson's helicopter nightmare a real possibility.

Increasingly, women like Susan Rogers want midwives to help them bear their children at home. With the reemergence of midwives in America today, it is important to ask why they ever disappeared.

As Dorothy and Richard Wertz point out in *Lying-In: A History of Childbirth in America,* physicians in the nineteenth century struggled to drive these women, their competitors, from the lying-in chamber. They saw midwives as threats to the very founding of their practice at a time when no established medical profession existed in North America. Women, they feared, might seek midwives for help with all their "female troubles," and doctors would lose at least half their potential patients.

BIRTHING IS LIKE A CAR CRASH

Historians emphasize this point: *Doctors did not replace midwives in America because their attendance at birth assured a safer outcome.* "They just claim that was the case, but it was not," says G.J. Barker-Benfield, assistant professor of history at the State University of New York at Albany and author of *The Horrors of the Half-Known Life,* a book that, in part, explores the origins of obstetrics and gynecology in America. "In fact, I'm trying now to explain the proliferation of gynecological disorders very often following birth at the hands of men. Contrary to being safer, obstetricians may well have been more damaging than midwives." The aggressive obstetrics of men, with the frequent use of forceps to speed up a labor process doctors often found tedious, lacerated cervices and tore holes in the birth canal. Professor Barker-Benfield noted.

During and after the antimidwife campaign, physicians redefined birth, changing it from a normal to a pathological process. They asserted that no precaution—including the employment of a physician—was too great to avoid its frightening dangers.

In 1920, an influential paper advocated routine forceps delivery and episiotomy (an incision made to widen the birth canal) for *all* deliveries. Dr. Joseph DeLee, one of the most revered men in American obstetrics, asserted that normal birth was pathologic and compared it to a baby's getting his head caught in a door.

Demonstrating that physicians still view birth as pathologic, Dr. Edward Hon, developer of the electronic fetal monitor (EFM), recently compared normal labor to a certain railroad crossing "where cars get smashed up and people get killed."

Such a dangerous event seemed to justify what obstetricians now call "active management of labor"—the artificial initiation, control, and termination of labor by doctors. This active management has gone far beyond the routine surgical procedure (episiotomy) that DeLee brought to normal birth, a procedure that has never been demonstrated, by any study, to benefit mothers or babies.

Interviews with prominent obstetricians reveal that by 2000, childbearing women (who under the pathological model of birth have become "patients") and their unborn babies can expect new forms of "active management."

Since obstetricians are developing techniques for reaching babies *in utero,* they may be peered at, medicated, and operated on before they are even born, several doctors enthusiastically told me.

In one procedure, the obstetrician will cut into the pregnant woman's abdomen and uterus and, using what is called a "fiberoptic endoscope," push into the amniotic sac and peer at the fetus through the telescopic lens in the instrument. Then the doctor will clip off a piece of the baby's skin and draw blood from it for what doctors call "diagnostic purposes."

Long-term effects of this procedure on mother and child are unknown; but Dr. R. Alan Baker, a fellow of the American College of Obstetricians and Gynecologists, lists some of the immediate risks to the mother.
• Spontaneous abortion.
• Leakage of amniotic fluid during later months of pregnancy.
• Uterine bleeding.
• Infection.
• Puncture of other organs.
• Rupture of the baby's blood vessels, leakage of

the blood into the mother's circulation, and the consequent buildup of antibodies in the mother against her child's blood.

• Psychiatric disturbances.

Baker questions whether fetoscopy — with its risks of uterine trauma, ruptured amniotic sac, damage to the eyes of the fetus from the intensity of the fiberoptic light — is a safe method of diagnosis. He points out that other, more accurate methods are available for determining congenital defects.

FETUS UNDER GLASS

In 2000, doctors will be able to medicate the "sick" fetus by injecting drugs into the amniotic fluid or by inserting a needle directly into the fetus. The success of the procedure, of course, will depend upon the doctor's ability to hit the right part of the unseen baby.

Long-term effects of injecting drugs into the still-developing fetus are unknown. However, testimony by Dr. Yvonne Brackbill, graduate research professor at the University of Florida in the departments of psychology and obstetrics-gynecology, before the Senate Oversight Hearings on Obstetrical Practices, in 1978, might give physicians cause for concern. Brackbill, who reviewed twenty-five students on the effects of obstetrical medication of the fetus, noted that the newborn is an organism poorly positioned for dealing with drugs. The drugs, she observed, "lodge in brain structures that are still developing and are therefore at high risk to damage. They are not readily transformed to nontoxic compounds since the necessary liver functionss are immature. And they are not readily excreted because of inefficient kidney function."

Obstetricians could, of course, peer at, medicate, and operate on a fetus more efficiently if it developed in a glass container. Even that is envisioned by one medical ethicist, Dr. Joseph Fletcher of the University of Virginia Medical School. During a discussion of the first test-tube baby, an ABC television interviewer asked Professor Fletcher last July, "Do you foresee the day when artificial wombs made of plastic or metal or whatever will be used?"

"Yes, yes, I foresee it with urgent approval," he replied. "I think I should be eager for the day when I could actually see, let's say through a glass container, a conceptus develop from fertilization through to term and see how all kinds of congenital mishaps which destroy or injure these babies might be prevented by medical tactics and medical strategies."

By 2000, electronic fetal monitors, used now to record the mother's contractions and the baby's heartbeat, may operate without wires, through telemetry (remote-control monitoring of a fetus), says Dr. L. Stanley James, of Columbia University, who specializes in the care of newborns. "That's the same as the astronauts have," he noted.

Dr. Edward Hon acknowledges that all the techniques for such monitors (key elements in the helicopter nightmare) are available today.

"There is a dual electrode that can be placed in the vagina right now," Dr. John Evrard, associate director of community reproductive health services at Women's and Infants' Hospital in Providence, adds. "And I foresee the time when we will have it transmitting to a piece of equipment while the woman is up and walking around. If they can do it from the moon to the earth, they certainly can do it from a woman to a console fifteen feet away."

(Space-age analogies come up extraordinarily often in conversations with obstetricians, indeed, obstetricians are already using technology developed in the space program.)

In the future, the monitors may be attached to digital computers. Referring to the development of this "computerized labor system," Dr. Charles Flowers of the University of Alabama School of Medicine wrote in an early paper on the concept that the project was designed "to utilize modern computer and electronic knowledge to monitor the fetus *in utero* with the same thoughtfulness as we monitor a man in space."

Dr. Saul Lerner, in a vision not shared by other obstetricians interviewed, hopes computers will calculate how long each stage of labor should be. In October 1977, Dr. Lerner, past president of the Massachusetts section of ACOG and a faculty member at the University of Massachusetts Medical School, told the *Boston Globe:* "We now have a very aggressive approach to pregnancy. There's a whole new concept plotted out by computers, how long each stage of labor should be. We will not allow a woman to labor for more than four hours without making progress. We do cesarean sections freely."

INTRODUCING THE BIRTH FACTORY

Acknowledging that hospital birth lacks "warmth," some doctors foresee a less mechanized birth by 2000. Obstetricians will develop machines and techniques that are unobtrusive, noninvasive, and less visible, they say. Surroundings will be made more pleasant for mothers. Curtains will be flowered.

"We'll be able to monitor things without too much invasion of the patient's body," Dr. Flowers of Alabama predicts. "We're going to combine warmth and a humanistic attitude with newer developments in electronics."

However, the fact that a regionalized system of perinatal care providing high-technology assistance for all pregnant women is now being established throughout the United States casts doubt on the prediction that birth will soon be rehumanized. According to a plan published in 1977, small maternity services in local communities will close down and all birthing mothers will be sent to large regional centers boasting the latest obstetrical technology.

Dr. Muriel Sugarman, a psychiatrist and a member of the Ad Hoc Committee on Regionalization of Maternity Services in Massachusetts, disapproves. The plan, she states, was devised by organized medicine, which believes ". . . that quality of care is measured by level of technological capability and that birth is a high-risk intensive-care, disease-ridden process on a par with cardiac surgery. . . ."

In the year 2000, Dr. Sugarman maintains, regionalized care will force mothers to go far from their communities and loved ones to bear their babies "in large, cold, impersonal birth 'factories.' "

Dr. Jack M. Schneider, codirector of what Dr. Sugarman might term a "birth factory"—the Wisconsin Perinatal Center in Madison—predicts that by the early 1980s, all pregnancies, registered by physicians with the regional perinatal center, could be monitored throughout the United States. Commenting on this prediction, Elliott M. McCleary writes in his book *New Miracles of Childbirth:*

"Then virtually every fetus nestled or kicking in every womb throughout America would have an electronic guardian angel in the form of a watchful computer."

Indeed.

It is this potential development, coupled with regionalization, that gives Suzanne Arms the same bad dreams Norma Swenson has. What it will take to realize the helicopter scenario, she thinks, is the implementation of regionalization "to the point where everybody knows what everybody else is doing."

The ability to "actively manage" birthing with the new technology gives obstetricians great power to control nature. Month by month, this power grows. As the world realized last summer with the birth in Britain of Louise Brown—conceived in a petri dish and delivered by a knife—doctors can control not only parturition (the birth process) but reproduction itself.

Physicians can artificially inseminate a

woman. They can fertilize an egg artificially. They can implant a fertilized egg in a uterus. Now men like Dr. Robert Goodlin of Stanford are hard at work on those glass or steel wombs whose mass production Dr. Fletcher so joyfully envisions. "Quality control" talk is on the increase.

Articles in the popular press now encourage parents to seek genetic counseling before they conceive, in order to prevent the production of "defective" children.

RETURN OF THE MIDWIFE

But perhaps reproduction and childbirth in 2000 will not be managed entirely as obstetricians would like it to be. A grassroots rebellion against establishment obstetrics is now beginning to gather momentum. It broke out, quietly at first, in 1960. Parents and childbirth educators, along with many nurses and some physicians, formed the International Childbirth Education Association. Respectfully, they challenged the validity of routine obstetrical practices and pressured obstetricians to adopt "family-centered maternity care." Under that program, husbands would be allowed to stay with their wives during delivery and women would be permitted to see their babies more frequently.

As the Protestants did, the movement is splitting into sects. In 1975, the National Association of Parents and Professionals for Safe Alternatives in Childbirth (NAPSAC) sprang up. The more militant NAPSAC members were not willing to ask physicians to "allow" them more participation in the birth of their children.

"We've done scientific research to determine what basis there is for hospital birth, and we don't find any basis," Dr. David Stewart, NAPSAC director, notes. "The only justification for going to the hospital is if you have some sickness or complication. This only applies to 10 or 20 percent of mothers." (His wife, Lee, delivered their children at home.)

Studies comparing home and hospital birth have found that for healthy mothers, the home is safer, Dr. Stewart, a physicist, continues. He refers specifically to studies by medical statistician Marjorie Tew and Dr. Lewis Mehl, director of research at the Center for Research on Birth and Human Development.

In 1972, other activists formed the Society for the Protection of the Unborn through Nutrition (SPUN). This group campaigns for scientific nutrition management in obstetrics and discourages obstetricians from prescribing the standard low-calorie, low-salt diet during pregnancy. Pointing to studies linking physician-supervised prenatal diets to serious disorders in the child and to toxemia in the mother, SPUN founders charge that the standard regimen — prescribed by obstetricians who have had no training in applied nutrition — damages the fetus.

In September 1977, SPUN won a precedent-setting case when a jury found an Indiana obstetrician guilty of malpractice for prescribing an inadequate diet and diuretics to a pregnant woman who subsequently gave birth to a mentally retarded child.

As SPUN, NAPSAC, and ICEA were growing, some women, rejecting expensive hospital maternity care they found dehumanizing, began to deliver their babies at home, often with the help of only a few inexperienced friends. These women began to be called upon for help by their friends and neighbors when they too wanted a home birth. They gained knowledge and skill. Some emerged as lay midwives.

In January 1977, more than 200 midwives held their First International Conference of Practicing Midwives in El Paso, Texas. "Home birth is a civil-rights issue." says Judith Luce, a lay midwife in Boston. "It's a woman's civil right to give birth where she chooses to give birth. It's a family's right to maintain the privacy of family life." Nationwide, an estimated 1.5 percent of births occur at home.

Such home-birth activists, who see obstetricians as a special-interest group, challenge the assumption that the values of physicians should be given more weight than their own. Their beliefs are generally summarized as follows: • Up to 90 percent of well-nourished childbearing women can give birth without difficulty or the need for obstetrical intervention. • Rather than continuing research on intensive-care units and sophisticated machinery for defective newborns, specialists in maternity care should emphasize the prevention of birth complications by counseling pregnant women on nutrition and by supplementing inadequate diets. • Obstetricians have an economic and emotional interest in suppressing midwives and in defining the needs of birthing women as highly complex. • As SPUN notes, major technological advancements in obstetrics and perinatology such as intensive-care nurseries, amniocentesis, and ultrasound have not led to marked improvement in maternal and infant health during the past two decades. (Amniocentesis entails inserting a needle into the uterus, drawing fluid from the amniotic sac of the fetus, and testing the fluid for metabolic and chromosomal defects. Ultrasound is a mechanical radiant energy used as an alternative to X rays to visualize the fetus. The external EFM also employs ultrasound in monitoring the fetus during labor.) • Many technological interventions in childbirth lead to iatrogenic (doctor-caused) illness. • The long-term effects of invasive diagnostic procedures and manipulations of normal labor (amniocentesis, elective induction of labor with oxytocin drugs, ultrasound, etc.) while as yet unknown, may be considerable and adverse. • They, as parents and their children will have to live with any adverse effects, and obstetricians will not.

As Dr. Stewart asserts, parents have a right to choose what may seem to the professional a wrong choice.

QUESTIONABLE PRACTICES

Childbirth organizations offer scrupulously documented critiques of many current obstetrical practices, the benefits of which, they maintain, have never been proven to outweigh their risks. They observe, as Dr. Lewis Mehl does, that standard obstetrical practices have often been established on the basis of single-case anecdotal reports that do not reflect systematic investigation and research.

Testimony presented at Senate oversight hearings on obstetrics last April supported Dr. Mehl's contention. Many drugs, surgical procedures, and instruments commonly used in obstetrics, Senator Jacob Javits stated there, had apparently "never been conclusively tested for the relative risk and benefit."

Dr. Donald Kennedy, Food and Drug Administration (FDA) commissioner, presented testimony that, while dispassionately phrased, constituted a devastating indictment of the unscientific way American obstetricians establish routine practices. In case after case, he reported that upon examination certain drugs and procedures widely used by obstetricians had been found: to be ineffective for the purpose to which obstetricians put it (DES and other synthetic hormones to prevent miscarriages: diuretic drugs to prevent toxemia; and, possibly, electronic fetal monitoring): • to expose mother and/or fetus to serious risks often to achieve an unclear benefit (elective induction of labor: X rays; sex hormones to diagnose pregnancy; pain-relieving drugs during labor; DES and other hormones for miscarriage; and electronic fetal monitoring, which, according to two studies, entails an increased risk of cesarean section without any improvement in infant outcome); • to present possible long-term effects, the extent of which obstetricians remain ignorant of (ultrasonic radiation and all of the above).

Senator Edward M. Kennedy observed at the hearings: "The development of obstetrical technology far outstrips our capacity to assess its appropriate value. As a result, common practice is established before appropriate practices can be defined."

The widespread use of ultrasonic equipment during pregnancy and in fetal monitoring during labor was a perfect example, he added. While ACOG believes ultrasound to be safe and recommends its widespread use, FDA scientists are concerned about its possible dangers, Kennedy noted. (In some animal studies, an increased incidence of fetal deformities has been found after low-level exposure to ultrasound.) EFM is another procedure widely used despite the fact that its efficacy has never been conclusively demonstrated. Developed in the 1950s by Dr. Edward Hon, now chief of perinatal research at University of Southern California Medical School, internal monitoring records fetal heart rate and uterine contraction pressure. The physician breaks the protective bag of waters prematurely and inserts two catheters containing electronic leads. One spiral electrode punctures the fetal scalp and relays the fetal cardiogram. The other relays the rate and pressure of uterine contractions.

Originally planned for high-risk pregnancies. EFM is increasingly being used routinely for *all* labors despite a study by Dr. J.F. Roux showing that one half the tracings of fetal heart rate and uterine contractions cannot be interpreted, that 25 percent of the women describe fear and pain associated with the monitoring catheter, and that complications include bleeding, minor vaginal and cervical lacerations, uterine perforation, increased incidence of infections, and fetal-scalp hematomas.

Moreover, a study by Dr. Albert Haverkamp of Denver General Hospital comparing the effectiveness of EFM to the old-fashioned method of monitoring fetal heart tones (with a fetascope) revealed no differences in infant outcome between the two groups. But there was a striking increase in cesarean sections performed for fetal distress in the electronically monitored group (16.5 percent versus 6.8 percent).

From 1971 until 1976 the cesarean-section rate increased 95 percent in the United States. The rate nationally is almost 20 percent of all births, and some doctors are arguing that it should go even higher.

Obstetricians assert that the rates are climbing because they are able to diagnose previously undetected "fetal distress" with EFM and save the baby through quick surgery. Dr. Haverkamp's study, and another conducted by a Harvard School of Public Health physician, challenges this belief. Moreover, Dr. Hon maintains that doctors are performing many unnecessary cesarean sections because they do not understand the meaning of the EFM tracings and they panic unnecessarily. "Most of the sections that are done for fetal distress are really done for obstetrician's distress," Dr. Hon has said.

For the mother, cesarean section is a major operation that always involves the risks of anesthesia and, sometimes, blood transfusion. Half the mothers suffer a post-operative complication.

Moreover, women have from five to twenty-five times greater risk of death from cesarean than from vaginal delivery. Despite such statistics, doctos are now routinely reaching for the scalpel at the first sign of irregular fetal-monitor indications.

OBSTETRICAL BACKLASH

Cindy Duffy, an Illinois woman who has had a cesarean, formed Cesarean Support to help others distressed by the operation. She notes that after the births of the 1940s and '50s, when women were often given the hallucinogen scopolamine, put out under general anesthesia, and not allowed to actively participate in the birth, mothers began insisting on "natural" childbirth. Thousands of mothers, she said, have since experienced rewarding births with minimal medical assistance. Now, many women are even delivering at home successfully.

"The obstetrician has seen his profession slowly lose its grip on women and made one last stab at regaining control via surgical interference," says Duffy. "After all, can you do a home cesarean?"

Ms. Duffy is not alone in sensing that obstetricians feel threatened by the growing home-birth trend. Shari Daniels, president of the National Midwives Association, believes the obstetrical establishment, in encouraging prosecution of midwives, is conducting a campaign to stamp out home births.

"In the next twenty years, I think a lot of us are going to have to go to jail," she says.

Citing a murder charge against a lay midwife and threats to dismiss an academician whose study placed a common obstetrical procedure in an unfavorable light, Dr. Stewart says of the obstetricians' campaign, "They mean for blood."

"It's a big-time economic issue," comments George Annas, associate professor of law and medicine at Boston University School of Medicine. "The number of children being born has gone way down and so has the census in obstetrical beds in hospitals. This is just another threat to obstetricians — that people are going to have their babies at home now. It costs them money every time somebody has a baby at home. That, I think, is the primary motivation behind the campaign against home birth."

Physicians, however, state that they oppose home birth because it endangers the lives of women and children. Dr. Edward Hon, who defines home birth as "child abuse," comments: "The dangers are so great with home birth that one wonders whether a woman has the right to make that decision for the unborn baby . . . we do not have a right to expose our minor children to undue hazard." Dr. John Evrard feels home birth is a "terrible mistake" and cites a January 1978 ACOG study showing a two to fives times greater infant mortality rate with out-of-hospital birth than with hospital delivery. The study is based on state health department statistics.

Dr. Stewart of NAPSAC contends that the ACOG study has confused out-of-hospital birth with home birth. The two are interchangeable terms since "out-of-hospital" birth statistics include miscarriages and premature births. He notes that the ACOG findings are not consistent with any other studies on home birth. In Holland, where, until recently, half the births occurred at home, the infant mortality rate was half that of the United States, he observes. Moreover, home-birth services in the US, including those run by the Chicago Maternity Center and the Frontier Nursing Service, have had excellent maternal and infant mortality rates.

The doctors' campaign against home birth, which appears to have gone into full swing in 1978, consists of actions against parents who participate in home birth and physicians, lay midwives, nurse-midwives, and childbirth educators who assist such parents.

According to Lee and David Stewart of NAP-SAC, obstetricians frequently refuse prenatal care and emergency backup to women who plan home births and, angry with women for having attempted home birth, verbally abuse those who are transported to the hospital. Health-department employees sometimes harass home-birth couples when they register the birth, they note.

In July 1977, ACOG's newsletter announced a registry of "preventable maternal deaths associated with home delivery."

"It is another example of obstetricians' collecting anecdotes and calling it science," Dr. Stewart commented.

Besides taking steps against couples who want out-of-hospital births, obstetricians have been pressuring birth attendants to cease their work in homes. Yale-New Haven Hospital in Connecticut has a policy of revoking the obstetric privileges of any staff physician who intentionally participates in a nonemergency home birth, *Ob-Gyn News* reported last January.

Other home-birth attendants, including May Blossom, a registered nurse in Ozark Hills, Missouri, have been charged with practicing medicine without a license.

A precedent for such charges was set in 1974 when police arrested lay midwives in Santa Cruz, California. Arguing that the charge against them—attendance at a normal physiologic function—did not constitute a crime, they refused to plead either guilty or not guilty. However, the State Supreme Court ruled that practicing midwifrey without a license is the same as practicing medicine without one.

The battle against midwives escalated when, last July, lay midwife Marianne Doshi was indicted for second-degree murder and practicing medicine without a license following the death of a baby at whose birth she attended. A California Superior Court judge subsequently dismissed the charges against Doshi. Judging from the medical testimony, he said, "I think the child would have died if it had been born in a hospital delivered by a doctor." He admonished the medical profession to have enough "maturity" to accept different birthing practices.

ILL-CONCEIVED LEGALESE

According to Suzanne Arms, author of *Immaculate Deception,* a bill to license midwives, introduced by California Assemblyman Gary K.

Hart, "addresses the basic issues of whether or not people have a right to choose the care givers that they want and whether these care givers have a right to appropriate high-quality training."

The original bill called for the development of midwives as independent healthcare providers for women in normal childbirth under the regulation of a Midwifery Examining Committee. After vigorous opposition from organized medicine, the bill was signed into law in September in a watered-down form that no longer mentions midwives specifically but rather "innovative health-care personnel."

Under the authority of the new law, though, the California Department of Consumer Affairs, which supports the licensure of lay midwives, reportedly plans to apply to sponsor a midwifery-training pilot project.

Shari Daniels, president of the National Midwives Association, would like lay midwives licensed throughout the country. In Texas, where she practices, midwives have asked that a Board of Midwives be set up, composed of midwives, consumers, and physicians. In most states now, she observes, the health department or the board of medical examiners would define standards for midwives.

"That means physical control," she points out. "It's like having Avis control Hertz."

Consumers and home-birth advocates are defending themselves somewhat from what they perceive as an obstetricians' campaign against them. In Illinois, members of Home Opportunity for the Pregnancy Experience (HOPE) have been working with state lawmakers to introduce legislation providing for the training and licensing of midwives. And last spring, Rhode Island passed legislation providing for state licensing of midwives.

At the Arizona School of Midwifery in Tucson, British midwives are now training fifty female students and preparing them to meet new state licensing requirements. The school, launched in 1977, is completely legal.

NAPSAC announced a "Clearinghouse for Legal Incidents Against Participants in Out-of-Hospital Birth" in 1978. By cataloging such actions, it would be able, if necessary, to counter "this assault" against conscientious parents and professionals engaged in home birth.

Despite such efforts, Attorney Annas notes: "Right now the obstetricians and pediatricians are organized across the country to oppose home birth. There's really been no concerted consumer movement against that. Parents don't have the interest in it that physicians have. They don't make their living doing that."

By 2000, most pregnant women will probably not participate in childbearing. The physician will "give birth" with his machines and knives. Thousands of renegade mothers, refusing to enter hospitals, will deliver their children at home, attended by midwives.

Obstetricians will wage battle against the midwives. They will hold fast to a tenet in the faith of Medicine. Every new technique represents progress. Doctors will continue to say that the operations they devise and the machines they invent (and sometimes hold patents on) perform socially laudable functions like saving lives.

Doctors will remain the same, but whether they will continue to enjoy the power they now hold depends in part on how the populace regards them. That, in turn, depends on the information people receive about medicine.

Will reporters who provide that information change in the next two decades and begin to demand evidence that these machines actually *do* what physicians say they do? Will they insist on examining reports of controlled studies that demonstrate a technique's efficacy and safety, and if no such studies exist will they report that fact? Or will they continue to write articles uncritically, glorifying technology and the miracles of modern medicine?

If so, the media will help doctors medicalize birth and shape the thinking of the populace.

And when Susan Rogers's neighbors hear that police forcibly took her to a hospital to have her baby delivered by knife, they will think it quite right.

THE CLONE DOCTOR

By William K. Stuckey

Up in the state of Vermont, in a town called Randolph, there's a good old country doctor who can take out my gizzard any day. His name is Landrum B. Shettles, and he knows more about bedside manner than anybody, even though he sometimes drops remarks that, as they say in his native Mississippi, "hit you right upside the head."

Doc Shettles got his gentle touch by doctoring ladies for thirty years, helping them with their female complaints and birthing their babies. Moreover, if they have trouble having their babies the usual way, he might just go and whip one up in a test tube. As a matter of fact, that test tube of Doc Shettles' might just put Randolph, Vermont, on the map, because he plans to use it to Xerox people with, if he doesn't get too many complaints, which I suspect he will.

Doc Shettles wants to be a cloner. Now, that

would be the biggest medical event to hit Randolph since 1841, when a healer named Jehiel Smith, who claimed he could cure people of all sorts of ailments by putting them in hot water with vegetables in it, accidentally made soup out of a fellow one day and had to leave town.

Doc Shettles and his associate, Dr. Romulo Valdez, would like to set up a fertility clinic right in Randolph, at the Gifford Memorial Hospital, if they can raise the money and don't get lynched. They would like to help women have babies, women who have blocked fallopian tubes and thus cannot conceive in the normal fashion. They would like to do this by mixing one of the woman's eggs with her husband's sperm in a test tube and then implanting the result in the woman's womb to complete the usual nine-month procedure. Doc Shettles thinks this is a good thing to do. As he puts it, "if the bridge is out, why not use a helicopter?"

If you have been reading the newspapers, you know that this technique of starting a baby in a test tube has been successfully accomplished both in England and in India. Doc Shettles claims he would have done it back in 1973 if his boss at Columbia University's Presbyterian Medical Center hadn't got upset and tossed the doc's test tube, contents and all, into the deep freeze.

As far as I can tell, the people in Randolph like Dr. Shettles and Dr. Valdez and generally approve of their plans for the fertility clinic. Of course, you can find one or two who wonder about that cloning business, even though it might be good for the local economy, what with all those rich tourists coming up to have themselves carbon-copied.

Doc Shettles is nobody's fool, but he likes to play little jokes on people, so you have to be careful about swallowing everything he says. (One Randolph resident remembers the time a lady brought Shettles a potted plant, and while she and the doc were having a serious conversation about gardening he took the plant out of the pot and replanted it upside down without batting an eye.) Nevertheless, I believed him when he told me that he knew how to clone people but would not do it except for the benefit of mankind. In other words, if you said, "Doc Shettles, I want you to make a full-fledged carbon copy of me, and here's the money," he wouldn't do it if he thought you were crazy, mean, wanted your name in the papers, or had carpetbagging tendencies. But I want you to decide whether or not he was telling me the truth on that fall day in Randolph, when the leaves were yellow as catfish eyeballs and as red as hog blood.

"You think a person ought to have the right to be cloned?" I asked.

"I think so," he said. "I feel that. If I wanted to be buried or cremated, that's my choice too, isn't it? Some people would rather be cloned than clubbed."

"You mean to tell me you'd attempt a cloning operation?"

"I wouldn't have any hesitation about it," he answered.

"You think it would work?"

"It'd be a lot of fun, and I'd try to make it successful. Why not?"

Of course, that "why not" of the doc's is a question as big a a particle accelerator, and if Shettles is telling the truth, and I think he is, he'll be spending the rest of his life answering it, as will his seven kids and the rest of us.

Now, cloning has been talked about for a long time, not only by such science-fiction writers as Arthur C. Clarke (in *Farewell to Earth,* for example) but also by such Nobel Prize winners as James Watson and Joshua Lederberg. And of course there was J. B. Gurdon, the English scientist who actually cloned a whole slew of identical frogs from the gut cell of a single frog. But Doc Shettles talks about cloning in a different way: He says it is easy to do. That's right, *easy.* If he's right, it won't be long before we see the neighbors coming home with Multiple Me kits.

I have to admit that I had little intention of talking about cloning when I went to see Doc Shettles in Randolph with my writer-daughter Marie (who is obviously no clone, because she is pretty). I went up to Vermont to see him about the Del Zio case, the recent trial in New York City that put the phrase "test-tube baby" on the front page of every newspaper in the country that was not then on strike. Shettles was an expert witness for Mrs. Doris Del Zio, who was suing Columbia University's Presbyterian Medical Center for the destruction of a test tube that she claimed contained her baby. Shettles was, in fact, *the* expert witness, for he had performed the *in vitro* fertilization that was to provide Mrs. Del Zio with the child she wanted.

Although Mrs. Del Zio won her case—she was awarded $50,000 in damages—Doc Shettles had been strongly criticized for his part in the whole affair and, he told me, was relieved to find that his patients in Randolph still liked him enough not to switch to another gynecologist. Still sensitive about all the things that were said about him during the trial, he showed me his *Who's Who* biography, his various awards and Phi Beta Kappa notice, as well as a number of letters from other doctors who said that he was far from being the biggest nut in the fruitcake. Mrs. Del Zio's lawyer had asked him to collect these documents and they were indeed impressive. One letter, from Dr. Houston Merritt, the former dean of the Columbia University College of Physicians and Surgeons, called Shettles "an excellent clinician and teacher and one of the foremost investigators in the country in the field of human reproduction . . . highly respected by his colleagues." (Shettles was on the staff at Columbia for twenty-six years.) Moreover, I couldn't help noticing from the journals and clippings that he was the first man ever to report the fertilization of a human-female egg outside of the body—that was in 1953—and also years ago made the discovery that there are two types of sperm, one carrying blueprints for a female and the other for a male. He also spent more than twenty years at Columbia with no complaints—that is, before his boss flushed his Del Zio project, and now he has a connection with nearby Dartmouth College's medical school.

And he is not one of those doctors ordained by

some California ten-dollar-diploma farm. Doc Shettles got his M. D. as well as a Ph.D. in cell genetics from Baltimore's famous Johns Hopkins Medical School. He's been to more places than Mississippi and Randolph, too, as you can tell from his memberships in several English medical groups with "Royal" in front of their names. Doc's paper collection also includes a 1973 letter from a big man in the National Institutes of Health saying that it is just as legal to do *in vitro* egg experiments in a test tube as it is to do *in lady* studies of the same subject. In other words, the Del Zio experiment was okay by Washington.

I was looking at him sideways while he was telling me all this, and I can tell you he is an interesting-looking man. He's about as high as a midget fence post, and he looks just as nice as your uncle, although some folks say he looks and talks like Truman Capote. He's still got that southern accent, which sounds a little funny there in Randolph, Vermont, and when he says "I don't know" it comes out "auno," but the Randolph folks don't hold that against him. Often his talk wanders around a bit, and trying to get his point is like trying to chase down a rabbit barefooted, but when he makes his point he does make it.

"You think that writer David Rorvik was telling the truth when he wrote that book *In His Image* claiming that a funny old millionaire had himself cloned back in 1976?" I asked.

"Well, I've been able to take the nucleus out of three human eggs and replace them with nuclei from the other body cells."

It might not sound to you as if old doc was answering my question, but he sure as Robert E. Lee was. What he was saying was that Rorvik was probably telling the truth, or at least that it was possible to take those first steps toward cloning a human person, because he, Doc Shettles, had taken those steps himself. Moreover, he had taken them since 1975, right there in his little down-the-block laboratory in Randolph, regardless of what the neighbors might think.

Now, getting more information from Doc Shettles on his country cloning was like pulling chicken teeth, because he wanted the official report of it to come out first in the *Journal of Obstetrics and Gynecology,* but then I found he'd already spilled some of his beans to America's finest backwoods science writer, old Charlie Siegchrist of Randolph's *White River Valley Herald.* (Shettles delivered Charlie's daughter.) So I figured it was all right to poke around a little more, and I did. But now you'll need a little science lesson on this—as I did—before you'll appreciate old doc's claims, and I promise not to make it hurt.

Now, your ordinary dive-bombing sperm cell has only twenty-three chromosomes in it, which sounds like a lot but is only half what you need to get a baby nine months later. Each one of those chromosomes hold about two yards of DNA, which stores up lots of information in little molecules for things like how big your brain is going to be, what color of skin you are stuck with, and even the shape of your toenails, as well as guarantees that you will be a human being, not a watermelon. What that sperm does when it meets a female egg is add its twenty-three to the egg's twenty-three, and when you get that magic forty-six the egg automatically begins to divide into all kinds of other cells, and you wind up with something that might look like you, me, or Landrum B. Shettles. Life has done it again.

Over there in Oxford and Cambridge, John Gurdon spooked the pants off all of us in the 1960s when he took out the nucleus of a frog's intestine cell and plopped it into a lady frog's egg cell that had had its nucleus pulled out, and that egg started dividing then and there, and, before you knew it, there was an exact croaking copy of that other frog who had had his gut played with. Gurdon had cut the boy frogs out of the whole sex act and did this over and over again. Before long, Doc heard about it and figured he'd try something like that with human eggs.

"You mean you went ahead and tried that with human eggs before testing the idea out in all kinds of other animals?" I asked.

"I started out with human-egg studies way back when almost everybody else was playing around with sea-urchin and rabbit eggs," he said. "I guess I've made more photographs of the human egg being fertilized and in its early stages of cleavage than anyone else alive, and those photos are hanging in science museums in New York, Boston, and other places. I don't like to work with laboratory animals like rats. The rats bite."

Now, I don't know if that was the real Landrum B. Shettles talking. I believe it could have been Landrum A. or Landrum C., or whichever one puts plants upside down in a flower pot. Anyway, he went looking for just the right cell with just the right forty-six, and he found it in the tissue involved in manufacturing sperm, which is pretty logical now that I think of it. Now you're going to say he cheated and slipped in one randy old sperm, but remember that sperm has only twenty-three chromosomes, while that sperm *maker* has the whole forty-six. The next thing Shettles did was to get an egg—Shettles doesn't say how he gets the eggs, but *New York* magazine once suggested he gets them any way he can and they called him an "egg poacher"—and suspend it in a mixture of fluids. All right, now Shettles faced the problem of how to get that sperm-maker nucleus out of its cell and into the poached egg. When Mr. Rorvik wrote his cloning book about that millionaire who wanted to be mimeo-graphed, he said that the high-powered doctors involved figured it was too hard to do nuclear transplanting by hand, so they used a virus to snip out the one nucleus and swim it into the egg. That is called the "fusion" method, as opposed to "microsurgery." But wait right there; Doc Shettles learned quite a bit about microsurgery way back in the thirties at Johns Hopkins, when he was sticking little glass needles into cells even without using that expensive automatic hand-steadying micro-equipment, since he and nobody else had any money then. What he said to himself was "I'm going to do this *free-hand,* and use my old Bunsen burner to make up a small, hollow glass pipette to go fishing for nuclei with," and he did. That would be quite a feat for anyone, especially for a man about seventy, and particularly when some Nobel Prize winners said it was too hard to do without damaging everything, since a human egg is much smaller than a frog's.

"I noticed in one of your testimonials that another big doctor complimented you for your 'fingers.' You must be pretty good with your hands," I said.

"Well, I grew up on a farm and I *was* good with my hands," he said. "I was a blacksmith and I was a carpenter, and one summer I fired the steam on a locomotive. I made a pipeline out of bamboo for an artesian waterworks. I studied at night by coal-oil lamp. When I was milking, I'd squirt milk right into a calf's mouth. Once, I trained a chicken how to catch corn."

Well, Doc Shettles made up his pipettes and went fishing, and three times, he says, he pressed a rubber bulb on the end of the pipettes and sucked out those sperm-maker nuclei and squirted them into those female eggs. Right before his eyes, those eggs not only began to divide, but divided six or seven times, producing a little pre-baby with some seventy or so cells. In other words, they were big and normal enough to transplant into a woman in test-tube-baby style.

Now, you have every right to ask whether the doc has any women lined up for ths part of his cloning operation, and he'll say he hasn't been looking for any and won't until the hospital gives him permission. But he suspects he won't have any trouble.

"You mean you've already had people ask you to clone them?" I asked.

"See this folder right here? It's about an inch and a half thick, isn't it? Well, it's got all the letters I've received since the Del Zio trial publicity, and maybe about fifty of them are asking me to help them have test-tube babies, and about half that number want me to try and reverse their tubal ligations, and, yes, I've got a few folks asking to be cloned. I have the facilities here to do anything I was able to do in New York."

"What are you telling them?"

"I tell them no for the time being," he said, "but that if things work out, I'll get in touch with them. I don't want to turn down any opportunities. Of course, I thought I might have had that opportunity back in 1975 when David contacted me."

"David? You mean David Rorvik?" I asked.

"I've known David since 1969, when he was writing for Time/Life," said Shettles. "He's written several articles about my work, and he helped me write that book *Choosing Your Baby's Sex,* and I can do that pretty good, although I doubt you want to hear about that now. I looked David in the eye, and I decided he had integrity. He wouldn't have done that cloning book for a stunt or for money if he hadn't thought it was the God's truth. Well, he wrote me back in June 1975 and told me about this cloning project. He said it involved a man from New Jersey, a millionaire in his mid-sixties, but he wouldn't give me his name, and he asked me for all the information I had on the subject. I sent him all the reprints I could find and made some sketches on how to do it with microsurgery, mentioning that I would immobilize the nuclei with carbon dioxide so that they wouldn't squirt around while I fished for them. However, I never heard from David after that, so I guess they decided microsurgery wasn't as good as the fusion approach. Of course, I don't know anything about fusion except for what I've read."

"Tell me one more thing," I said. "What if a woman wanted herself cloned and wanted to use her own egg holding her own transplanted forty-six chromosome body cell, and wanted to stick it back in and carry it herself for the nine months? Would that work?"

"I hadn't thought about it," he answered. "I don't see why not, though. I bet you're going to tell people I'm a mad person. When you get older, you begin to think on things. I could go just like that. I try to appreciate today. I don't want to sound morbid, but I don't think I'm any unhappier by thinking about the different ramifications of life, such as cloning. Why not? I'd just like to see if it would work. Of course, there might be some unforeseen ramifications."

Well, before I did too much head work on those unforeseen ramifications, I thought I'd take a walk around Randolph and admire those colored leaves and white church spires, and dropped into Wesley Hurwig's Randolph Historical Museum, where I found out that Randolph had been named for the first chairman of the Continental Congress back in 1776 and barely missed becoming Vermont's capital in 1805. I wandered around, staring at some of the honest faces of the 4,500 Randolphians, who work mostly at making wood and dairy products, but who also make plastics, tools and dies, and work gloves. And if Doc Shettles has anything to do with it, there might be a new type of manufacturing industry in Randolph soon.

I visited over the kitchen table with Mrs. Edna Braun, a former mental-health worker, who said that Shettles is lovable, tolerant, kindly, and sharp as a tack, even though it might be a slightly odd-shaped tack. She thinks he ought to be let alone to work, even though she is an Irish Catholic from Boston and the pope back in 1954 condemned the type of work that Shettles did. I talked to Tom Rogers, the controller of a local bank and solid citizen if there ever was one, who likes Doc just fine, although he holds back a little from giving Shettles's cloning desires a flat-out endorsement. Everywhere I went, I was told that Randolphers are a levelheaded but conservative folk who take years to warm up to outsiders and newcomers, but that they accepted Doc right off when he moved up from New York in 1975 to get away from that high overhead that was keeping him from helping people in his *own* way. Charlie Siegchrist himself told me that when his story came out in the *White River Valley Herald* on March 9, 1978, it was talked about a lot in the Rainbow Café, but nobody got too excited about it or went for the tar and feathers or anything. Randolphers generally believed it wasn't their business, and a fellow ought to mind his own business even if it is a funny one.

The main thing to remember about Shettles though is that it really doesn't make much difference what he does in the cloning way if he is right about the other part—that it is a fairly easy thing to do. Remember how there never had been any heart transplants until that South African fellow did it one day in the 1960s, and before you knew it, everyone was doing it? And of course as far as we know, the Russians, the Chinese, and old Howard Hughes might have already done some cloning, if not a lot of it; and we've already heard what David Rorvik claims. Naturally, it gives me pause, as I don't know just how many more of me I could stand, not to mention not being needed to start off the whole daddy business anymore. Now, how would I feel if I were a clone? Could my "daddy" or "mama" claim I was a piece of property with no constitutional rights, the same way some folks have patented certain types of cloned grain or plant seeds or farm animals? Now, wouldn't there be some folks who would claim I wasn't really human, even though I felt as if I was? And wouldn't at least some of them want to wipe me out, as has been done to "different" or "inferior" races over the years? And wouldn't I want to wipe them out in self-defense? As a matter of fact, if you throw in what we'll probably be facing with computers in a few years, won't folks all over the world become downright confused over what being "human" is? If it is true that different types and races of folks breed stronger children when they get together behind the barn, as the old folks claim, and if you get ones that are weak in the head when people too much alike, like cousins, intermarry, then what can you expect the result to be if someone makes his children from his own liver? If this cloning really gets to be serious business, I imagine that some countries are going to go and start passing laws controlling reproduction among the taxpayers — especially among those with no political clout.

After a while I went on back to Gifford Memorial Hospital to say good-bye to Doc Shettles, but before he let me go, he took me around to see some of his egg photos, which he has taken in almost thirty years of being a laboratory-camera nut. There was one with two sperm cells crossed over one another — one a boy sperm and the other a girl. They were, as the English heraldry experts say, rampant upon a field of Egg.

"I call this one 'Man's coat of arms,' but you'll note that the ladies make up two thirds of it," said Doc Shettles.

"I think you ought to be cloned," I answered.

"No, no, no," he said. "You know, once my daughter asked me if I believed in reincarnation, and I said I didn't know, and she said that if there was any such thing, I'd come back as a squirrel."

Way up there in Randolph
There's a sight you ought to see.
That good old country cloner
Is Xeroxin' you and me.

I'M CLONED, I'M CLONED, I'M CLONED!
I'VE GONE TO GLORY NOW!
But since there's all those Me's around,
It's all the same somehow.

PART SEVEN:
PATHWAYS TOWARD PROGRESS

I SING THE BODY ELECTRIC

By Kathleen McAuliffe

Imagine if we could speak to cells, instructing them to grow more quickly or slowly, change their shape and function, or organize themselves into new tissues to replace damaged ones. Without lifting a scapel to flesh or injecting a chemical into the bloodstream, scientists are doing just that. They have discovered a way to tap into the body's internal communication network and transmit messages in a language that cells understand. That language consists of electrical signals—the universal code by which living organisms regulate growth, development, and repair.

We all wear an invisible garment, an electromagnetic cloak that shields us from head to toe. From the moment of conception, electrical currents begin to flow in the tiny embryo, guiding the incredibly intricate process that culminates in birth. When a salamander regrows a limb, similar currents flow along the injured extremity as if re-enacting a crucial step of embryo-genesis. Once the new organism — or limb — is fully formed, the currents abate. Yet we all retain an electromagnetic halo as a birthday suit that we carry throughout life. Disturbances in these fields portend illness. In fact, this is the basis of acupuncture diagnosis. Whenever bodily injury is sustained, our primordial durrents flow strong until the wound heals over.

Bioelectricity is nothing new. As far back as the eighteenth century, Luigi Galvani discovered this source of energy in the twitching of a frog's leg strung between two pieces of metal. Only recently, however, have we realized just how pervasive a role electricity plays in governing vital cellular functions. Our enlightenment has revealed a radical new approach to medical therapy: Doctors are seeking to alter our internal currents with external ones. By applying electricity to the body, they believe, it will one day be possible to grow back the amputee's limb, repair the paraplegic's severed spinal cord, and stop the cancer victim's uncontrolled proliferation of cells.

"Electricity will become as ubiquitous in medical practice as surgery or drugs; in many instances it will supplant them," says Dr. Andrew Bassett, of Columbia-Presbyterian Medical Center, in New York City. An orthopedic surgeon, he was one the first to use electricity to mend bone fractures that had stubbornly resisted all other treatments. Dr. Bassett's technique is to position electric coils around the injury so that a pulsating electromagnetic field induces tiny currents in the bone.

"The patients love it," Bassett says, "because they don't have to go under the knife." They don't even have to be hospitalized. Once the coils, given out only by prescription, have been specially fitted, they can be taken home in a lightweight case. If they are worn 12 hours a day, the fracture usually mends within four to six months. And the therapy is totally painless.

"You would experience almost the same field strength by standing under a fluorescent light," Bassett says, "except that the fields employed in therapy are organized in a different informational pattern."

BEYOND BONE REPAIR

So far, bone healing is the only use of his electrical coils approved by the U. S. Food and Drug Administration, but Bassett is anxious to see the applications spread beyond the orthopedic wards. From his animal studies, for example, Bassett discovered that electricity will consistently double or triple the growth rate of peripheral nerves—those found in the limbs.

"If peripheral nerves are severed," says Bassett, "they rarely repair themselves. If an individual ruptures his sciatic nerve in a head-on collision or puts his hand through glass and cuts his median nerve, years of therapy may be required before he regains even a fraction of the normal motor control."

Although only two human patients have been

tested up until now, Bassett is greatly encouraged by the results: The electromagnetic field promoted the same beneficial nerve growth seen in laboratory animals. "It's still too soon to say whether this is the panacea for peripheral nerve injuries or not," Bassett cautions. "Time will tell. But I think we have the upper edge."

It is clear Bassett believes that electricity will also give medical science the "upper edge" in repairing damage to the central nervous system. A solution to this pressing problem might benefit more than 6 million people in the United States alone, ranging from paraplegics to stroke victims.

How does electricity produce these startling effects? Cells respond to artificially induced currents just as well as to the body's own. Nature alone performs miracles; scientists merely exploit them.

Earlier in this century several investigators began to study the electrical currents produced by a variety of living organisms—from embryonic seaweed to tadpoles. Working after World War II, Dr. Robert O. Becker, of the Veterans Administration Hospital in Syracuse, New York, had one distinct advantage over his predecessors: the growth of sophisticated electronic technology. "The kinds of tools available to me right off the shelf were much more sensitive," Dr. Becker said. Although many of his colleagues see him as the supreme catalyst in the field—"the man in modern times who asked the right questions at the right moment," one puts it—Becker takes another view: "If you look at things from a historical perspective, I'm not such a smart guy. I was just plain lucky."

Becker's involvement in electrical therapy began with a pioneering study of injury currents. Immediately after an organism is wounded, damaged cells become leaky. Charged atoms, called ions, pour out of the cells, forming a current. By measuring voltages generated at injury sites, Becker uncovered clues to one of nature's most baffling inequities: why the lowly salamander can regenerate as much as one third of its total body mass, while man can scarcely endure damage to a single vital organ. Moreover, his findings suggested that currents of only a few billionths of an ampere might be the key to rectifying this gross imbalance of the evolutionary scale. Using an implanted electrode, Becker stimulated a rat to regrow its amputated foreleg down to the elbow joint. The portion that grew back was not perfect, but there was clear evidence of multitissue organization, including new muscle, bone, cartilage, and nerve.

Then a researcher at the Univeristy of Kentucky Medical School, Dr. Stephen Smith, applied the same technique to regenerating the legs of frogs. A more highly evolved species than the salamander, the frog cannot normally grow back an amputated extremity. But Dr. Smith modified Becker's procedure in one important way. Electricity was introduced through an electrode that migrated down the limb as new tissue grew back. "In one instance," he reported, "a new leg formed in complete anatomical precision, right down to the individual digits of the frog's webbed feet."

For over 20 years Becker has doggedly pursued an unorthodox theory: Higher animals — whether frog, rat, or man — don't naturally regenerate limbs because they produce too little electricity to trigger the formation of a limb bud. Becker has long suspected that, given the appropriate electrical environment, the cells in our body — like those in the salamander — could still be made to differentiate into new tissues.

"It is time the medical establishment accepted the concept that a considerable amount of regenerative growth could be restored to the human," he states in his characteristically forthright manner. "This applies to almost every tissue in the body, from the brain through the spinal cord to peripheral nerves, fingers, whole limbs, and organs. Of we can identify the mechanisms that stimulate and control regeneration in the salamander, I see no innate reason why man cannot be stimulated to do the same thing."

MIRACLES IN THE MARROW

If the "medical establishment" has been slow in coming round to his viewpoint, it is hardly astonishing. Until Becker's landmark experiment on the rat in 1973, many doctors considered his ideas heretical. That weak currents could transform an amputee's stump into a limb seemed more akin to witchcraft than to medicine. Furthermore, Becker's theory assumed that mammalian cells were capable of extraordinary feats, for the process of regeneration is, in its very essence, a rebirth.

When a salamander regrows a limb or an organ, red blood cells at the injury site lose their specialized function. They return to a primitive, almost prenatal state, ready to be molded anew. In fact, this cluster of amorphous cells is called a blastema, a term sometimes applied to embryonic cells. As the blastema grows in size, the undifferentiated cells become specialized again, regrouping themselves into all the complex tissues of the body part that they are to replace.

No one ever dreamed that mammalian cells could undergo such a dramatic metamorphosis. For a start, our red blood cells, unlike those of the amphibian, have no nuclei and thus do not contain genetic material. Yet when minute electrical currents were applied to the rat's forearm, a blastema formed. Becker's detective work soon solved this mystery. In mammals, the blastema appears to be derived from nucleated cells in the bone marrow.

The implications were far-reaching: We have retained our ancient ancestors' capacity to regenerate! It is only the controlling factor that has been lost over the course of evolution. All the evidence pointed to electricity as the controlling factor, but a central enigma remained. Why do some organisms generate more than others? What drives the injury current?

Acupuncturists have long been aware of electromagnetic fields surrounding the body. Eastern practitioners today commonly monitor variations in these fields to diagnose underlying disease. In his effort to track down the "organic battery" that powers the injury current, Becker began to investigate these natural fields. Over a five-year period he measured stable voltages on the skin of organisms ranging from the salamander to man. In all instances the fields roughly paralleled the major pathways of the nervous system.

This gave Becker an important lead, for a mysterious link between nerves and regeneration had been known since the early 1950s. Dr. Marcus Singer, at Case Western Reserve University, in Cleveland, showed that nerves must make up at least one third of the total tissue mass in an extremity before regeneration will occur spontaneously. By transplanting extra nerves to a frog's forelimb, he produced about a centimeter of new tissue growth at the amputation site. Could nerves provide the electrical signal that triggers blastema formation?

To find out for sure, Becker carried his investigation one step further. He measured electrical voltages on the outside of the nerve fibers themselves. According to standard textbook accounts, there is only one mechanism by which nerves transmit an electrical signal. That message consists of a series of brief impulses that move down the nerve fiber. Becker, however, discovered what he believes to be a second and more primitive method for the nervous system to transmit information. His measurements indicated that the cells coating the outside of peripheral nerves carry a continuously flowing current, in contrast to the short bursts of electrical activity the nerves themselves conduct. This constant current, he believes, radiates throughout the body's dense network of peripheral nerves and gives rise to the field patterns all organisms display. It seemed logical to him that disturbances in these fields, created by an injury, for example, would be detected by cells, which would then begin repair processes. If the nerve mass were large enough, the voltages generated could be sufficient to initiate complete regeneration. Otherwise, scar tissue would form.

Becker's theory clashed with the traditional concept of how the nervous system functions. "I got an awful lot of lumps on my head when I first published my report in *Nature*," he recalls. But his colleagues' initial skepticism has gradually given way to broader — although by no means universal — acceptance.   Neurophysiologists, Becker reports, have been the most receptive to his ideas.

Although there are nonbelievers at a theoretical level, few doubt the practical significance of Becker's work. A growing number of scientists are now confident — which scientists weren't only a decade ago — that regeneration of human body parts will be achieved, probably within our lifetime. And it was Becker, in conjunction with Bassett, who developed the electrical method of healing bone fractures. The treatment may earn both doctors a Nobel Prize in medicine. (It has been rumored that Becker's name appeared on the Nobel committee's list of nominees last year.)

ION MESSENGERS

Bone healing is one of the few examples of man's ability to regenerate an injured part spontaneously. "It is truly a regenerative process," says Becker, "because a blastema actually forms." In this instance, however, the source of electrical voltage is not the nerves alone. The bone itself becomes electrically polarized when bent or broken. As Bassett and Becker discovered, its crystalline structure converts mechanical stress into electrical energy — a finding independently made at about the same time by two Japanese doctors, Iwao Yasuda and Eiichi Fukada. These voltages in turn help to guide cellular-repair mechanisms, beginning with the appearance of a blastema at the fracture site. Unfortunately, sometimes something goes awry in the normal healing process and a troublesome nonunion develops. Electricity, they reasoned, might be the solution.

Animal studies confirmed the idea. Then, by introducing direct current through an electrode at the fracture, Dr. Carl Brighton and his colleagues at the University of Pennsylvania Medical School were able to cure severely crippled patients, many of whom had been scheduled for amputation because their disabled limbs had become infected. At dozens of clinics in the United States and abroad, electricity has become the preferred treatment for difficult bone nonunions. Since the first clinical experiments, however, orthopedists have varied in their approach to electrotherapy. Bassett, for example, prefers electrical coils to electrodes because they preclude surgical intervention. His procedure's success rate is 85 percent; he hopes it will eventually work in 95 to 98 percent of cases.

RELIEF IN SPACE

Bassett's coils are so simple to operate that astronauts may use them in space to prevent what NASA officials commonly refer to as astro-osteoporosis. Astronauts' bones become thin and brittle owing to a loss of calcium. Over prolonged space missions, the condition worsens. When the Soviet cosmonauts first returned from their 175-day journey aboard *Salyut 6,* they were no more capable of walking than jellyfish are. Vigorous rehabilitation is required to recover from this "spaceman's disease," which for a while threatened to jeopardize the future of manned space exploration.

But astro-osteoporosis is not a disease. In fact, it is a remarkable adaptation to life in zero gravity. "The astronauts produced less bone," says Bassett, "because they didn't need big, heavy bones in the weightlessness of space. Their bone was under less mechanical stress. Hence, it did not generate the normal electrical voltages that help maintain bone formation." The coils, he believes, should counteract what would otherwise be a superior adaptation to permanent residence in space.

Like several other doctors in the forefront of electrical medicine, Bassett is now attacking the problem of repairing damage to the spinal cord—the cause of partial or total body paralysis. Earlier in his career, while working with neurosurgeon James B. Campbell, he discovered a simple, nonelectrical technique to promote central-nervous-system growth. After the scientists created a defect in a cat's spinal cord, the injured area would be wrapped in a millepore sleeve, a type of filter material. Hundreds of thousands of nerve fibers would grow across the gap.

"Unfortunately," says Bassett, "the lower half of the cat's body remained paralyzed. By the time the nerve fibers had grown back, the motor neurons below the point of transection had formed abnormal connections with neighboring cells — what we call collateral sprouting. The switchboard was busy. There were no free circuits for the nerves to connect to.

"Now what triggers collateral sprouting in the first place is an injury current. To open the switchboard, we then inserted electrodes into the spinal cord. This drove the voltage in the opposite direction, countering the injury current. In fact, we found we could eliminate collateral sprouting in small, defined areas. To do this on a practical basis, however, we would have needed two billion electrodes, each touching an individual cell. But now we can induce currents in the spinal cord using coils. We don't have to make do with electrodes."

DOGGED EXPERIMENTATION

Bassett has a commanding presence. Behind his facade of determination one senses a warm man who has much compassion for his patients. While we were sitting in his office, one of his experimental subjects — a short-haired beagle — arrived for his inspection. Surrounding its head was a fan-shaped collar, lending the animal the majestic air of an Elizabethan grande dame. The beagle, which Bassett greeted affectionately, had just undergone an experiment studying the effects of electricity on wound healing. The collar prevented the dog from licking the open sore.

"What sore?" I asked, looking over the dog's shiny pelt.

"Well, as you can see, the experiment was successful," Bassett said. "Depending upon the electrical fields we apply, it is possible to modify the pattern of wound healing." Very shortly he will be launching clinical studies to see whether the same approach can be used to heal bedsores, which afflict 20 to 30 percent of all invalids.

Equally encouraging, Drs. Walter Booker and E. B. Chung, at Howard University, in Washington, D. C., have been very successful in treating burn victims with pulsed electromagnetic fields. The therapy not only accelerates healing but reduces swelling around the charred flesh. Dr. Chung says, "Patients report almost immediate relief after a single therapeutic session."

A recurrent pattern pervades the history of medicine: Often new treatments are adopted long before anyone fully understands why they work. Electricity is no exception. Becker's meticulous probing has helped to identify several important sources of bioelectricity, from the electrical voltages generated by bone to the electromagnetic fields that radiate from our nerve network. Yet there is an aura of mystery around the magical transformations that take place at the most fundamental level—that of the cell. By intercepting the electrical messages the body transmits, scientists have learned how to code signals that make sense to cells. In effect, they are practicing a form of speech through mimicry—without understanding the basis of the language itself. What information is encoded in the electrical signal? Why do cells alter their behavior in response to changes in their electrical environment?

CELLULAR FINE-TUNING

There are still many more questions than answers, but a few unifying principles have emerged. In an office adjacent to Bassett's, electrochemist Art Pilla develops and fine-tunes the electromagnetic pulses used in therapy. "In every single living system studied," Pilla says, "we have found that the same level of currents is required to exert cellular control. If the amplitude and frequency of the electromagnetic current do not fall within a specific range, cells fail to respond." Only when he tunes the signal into the "biological waveband" is it possible to establish a dialogue with cells.

In cellular communication, ions—not words—are the key elements. "At the right waveband," Pilla explains, "the electrical signal appears to move ions, such as sodium, magnesium, and calcium, across the selective membrane of the cell. This in turn unleashes a chain of chemical reactions within the cell itself, which may ultimately lead to the unraveling of DNA—the first step toward growth and repair." According to Pilla, the influx of ions may determine, among other things, why some genes are switched on or off. Could electricity transform a cancerous cell into

350

a normal one? Or a bone cell into cartilage? Pilla is seeking the answers to these and other questions that are inextricably tied to genetic control.

Unlike other pioneers in this new field, Pilla did not originally train in biological science. Before he joined the research team at Columbia-Presbyterian, he worked for a battery manufacturer. Then, while flying to the West Coast to attend a conference on electrochemistry, he happened to sit beside a member of Bassett's group.

Today, almost 12 years later, Pilla is convinced that electricity is a revolutionary technique for controlling innumerable processes in the body. "I've always believed in a Morse code approach," he says. "That we could, in fact, send in heavily coded signals and modulate everything. Of course, we don't know how to do it yet!" he exclaims. "But that day is approaching."

Sitting at his computer console, working out the pulsed wave forms he uses, Pilla has the gleeful look of a young child who has just been given a new toy. His enthusiasm is contagious. Dozens of scientists consult him daily over the phone, and he is always entering research projects with them. Every time he gets his hands on a new piece of information, it sparks off yet another idea for an experiment. Working in collaboration with Smith, he has helped develop electrical pulses that will speed salamander limb regeneration by a factor of four—or stop new tissue growth altogether. "In the presence of some fields," says Pilla, "the salamander looks as if it is a nonregenerating form."

CANCELING CANCER

Smith and Pilla are also studying the effects of electricity on cancer growth. "We have found certain pulses that kill lymphoma cells grown in culture," Pilla remarks. "Other fields change the cell lining of the lymphoma, transforming it into a fibroblast—a type of connective-tissue cell found throughout the body."

Both scientists caution that their research is still merely at the experimental stage. Yet they are optimistic about the results of one of the first animal studies, which Pilla conducted with William Riegelson, of the Medical College of Virginia, and Larry Norton and Laurie Tansman, of Mount Sinai School of Medicine, in New York City. At the one hundred fifty-seventh meeting of the Electrochemical Society, held in St. Louis last May, the team reported that mice injected with deadly melanoma cells lived an average of 27 days when untreated, 36 days if given chemotherapy, and 43 days when chemotherapy and electricity were combined. Though these early findings are encouraging, more research will be required before electricity's true potential in cancer therapy can be properly evaluated. Pilla notes that the electrical pulses will probably have to be refined for each individual, depending upon the type of cancer.

Cancer therapy is far from the only exciting avenue of research Pilla is now pursuing. He is equally intrigued by the possibility of using electromagnetic fields to alter brain functioning. To test his theories, he is now working with Dr. Ross Adey, president of the Veterans Administration

Hospital in Los Angeles. Bassett describes Dr. Adey as "one of the most amazing individuals in biophysics today." Adey has shown that he can increase the rate of learning and memory retention in primates and cats by focusing an electromagnetic field at the animal's head while training is under way. The electrical signal is carried over a radio frequency, and Adey modulates its amplitude in the same way an AM radio is tuned. Adey believes that neurological changes occur because the frequency of the electrical signal is within the same range as the alpha and beta waves of the brain. But Pilla emphasizes another interesting aspect of his results. He thinks Adey's findings represent a more general phenomenon: The currents he uses to enhance learning and memory just happen to be similar to those that are biologically active in other cell systems.

For the immediate future, most experts agree that electrical therapy will have the greatest impact in healing tissues that do display some regenerative capacity—skin, bone, and peripheral nerves. But as science becomes more sophisticated in controlling vital functions with electricity, infinite possibilities may open up. Conquering cancer, regrowing whole limbs and organs, and augmenting the brain's cognitive processes are just a few of the advances that electrical medicine may offer.

Earlier in this century the introduction of vaccines and antibiotics brought enormous improvements in the treatment of smallpox, scarlet fever, tuberculosis, and other infectious diseases. Electricity may bring about a comparable revolution in the treatment of chronic diseases and physical impairments now thought beyond hope. "There is not a single branch of medicine that will remain unchanged as a result of this powerful tool for controlling life processes," Bassett declares.

AGENT X

By Franklynn Peterson
and Judi Kesselman-Turkel

Restless and ravenously hungry, the killers fanned out in search of living food. Their goal: to invade the body of any healthy organism, capturing its life-force for the production of still more lethal agents.

Conceived by science-fiction writer Ralph Milne Farley in a 1936 story entitled "Liquid Life," the gelatinous monsters were minuscule, viruslike mutants that matched humans in intelligence. They were able to pass through filters fine enough to trap all known viruses. And the only chemical that could destroy them was carbolic acid.

Today 200 researches throughout the world are racing to unravel the mysteries of a *thing* that could have stepped right out of Farley's fantasy. This thing is also a deadly mutant that passes through filters fine enough to trap all known viruses; it appears to be vulnerable only to carbolic acid. Scientists call it viroid, viruslike agent, scrapie agent, and other names just as vague. We'll call it Agent X.

A brutal but insidious murderer, Agent X enters living organisms, settling happily in and causing no trouble for years. Then suddenly it strikes with a vengeance that has jarred medical science. Victims first become too dizzy to walk, then too ill to stand. Their thought processes gradually slow until they seem senile or demented. In a year they are dead.

So far Agent X has been detected in nature only in sheep, minks, and humans—particularly one New Guinea cannibal tribe. Because it has been so elusive, scientists suspect it might be the cause of a wide range of unexplained debilitating diseases: multiple sclerosis, rheumatoid arthritis, and even diabetes. It cannot be cured by interferon, radiation, or any of the virus and bacteria killers devised by man.

Until the discovery of Agent X, the ordinary virus was the tiniest known organism. Smaller than a single human cell, it consists merely of a strand of nucleic acid (a gene) surrounded by a protein shell. Without the protein-synthesizing machinery found in other living cells, the virus can neither grow nor reproduce. So, like Farley's fantastic little particle, it perpetuates by invading other living organisms, using their cellular machinery to manufacture more virus.

Agent X *seems* to reproduce in much the same way. However, scientists scrutinizing its structure can find no protein shell and no trace of nucleic acid, the building block of genes in every other form of life. Agent X cannot be classified: It is not really a virus, but rather a bizarre mutant that changes form from one generation to the next. Almost impossible to detect, it is so tiny that 1 billion particles could fit on the head of a pin one millimeter in diameter. The same pin could hold a third as many polio viruses. Researchers on the track of this ruthless scavenger expect they will eventually have to broaden, or even redefine, terms like *virus* and *gene*. When they do, they may have to draw up a new definition of life.

Agent X can be traced back to 1755, when English sheep farmers petitioned Parliament for relief after massive numbers of sheep died from scrapie, so called because the sheep first showed signs of the illness by scraping against posts and rocks, apparently to relieve itching. Later they lost the ability to walk, and still later their sense of balance was so disrupted they couldn't even stand. Scrapie symptoms appeared most often in the third year of a sheep's life and usually killed the animal before it was four years old. Today scrapie is known to be caused by Agent X.

A nineteenth-century scrapie epidemic in Germany was considered the agricultural equivalent of the black plague. By the early 1950s scrapie had become too costly a killer to be ignored, taking 1 sheep out of about every 100. So in several countries agriculture departments began eradication campaigns.

To wipe out a disease, you generally must know what's causing it. But by 1954 scientists knew only that scrapie was transmitted from animal to animal *somehow,* by *something.* Because sheep didn't show scrapie symptoms until the third year, scientists named the causative "thing" *slow virus.* Later it was pointed out that minks with a disease called transmissible mink encephalopathy (TME) showed similar symptoms. TME, too, was attributed to slow virus, again pretty much on the basis of a scientific hunch.

Back then scientists were relatively certain that scrapie couldn't spread through the air, in water, or by chance contacts, which are normal routes for viral infections. They suspected that scrapie got around only by direct, intimate contact, for example, when a healthy sheep ate a placenta left behind by a diseased sheep. This was effectively confirmed when Richard Marsh, a veterinarian at the University of Wisconsin demonstrated that TME and scrapie were one of the same disease and that minks caught it by eating scraps of scrapie-infected sheep.

Then, in 1957, an American pediatrician named Carleton Gajdusek stumbled onto the trail of Agent X while visiting a friend in New Guinea. Gajdusek, an intense young man with piercing brown eyes and a rapid clip to his speech, met a district medical officer who told him about a strange neurological disorder. It was found only among the Fores, a group of cannibals, the officer said. The disease, called kuru, killed about 1 in every 100 Fore people, mostly women and children. The stricken were first unable to walk, then unable to talk or even see. They sank into a world of madness and confusion, and inside of a year they were dead.

So fascinated was Gajdusek that he stayed in New Guinea for a year, trading axes and tobacco for the tissue remains of kuru victims. He was able to prove that kuru chewed the brain to a spongy pulp, especially the cerebellum, which controls motor function. But nowhere could he find the elusive particle of destruction. In 1958 he accepted a post as visiting scientist at the National Institutes of Health (NIH), in Bethesda, Maryland, and started publishing his findings.

One of Gajdusek's papers was read by William Hadlow, a veterinary scientist who had spent most of his career tracking down scrapie. Hadlow, with NIH's Rocky Mountain Laboratory, in Montana, quickly recognized the extraordinary similarity between kuru and scrapie. In a letter to *The Lancet,* he made the brave leap to the theory that both diseases were caused by the same mysterious agent.

Following Hadlow's suggestions. Gajdusek spent years observing the lab chimpanzees he had inoculated with homogenized brain tissue from kuru victims. In 1963, a few years after the inoculations began, the first chimps developed kuru, and Gajdusek concluded that the disease could be transmitted from one animal or person to another. Convinced that the Fores passed along Agent X via cannibalism, Gajdusek persuaded them to end the practice. Now the disease no longer strikes members of the tribe.

Because kuru was a cannibals' disease, it received more attention than the sheer number of victims would have warranted. But Gajdusek soon learned that another, far less publicized neurological disorder — Creutzfeldt-Jakob disease (CJD) — had markedly kurulike symptoms. Victims lost the ability to walk or talk, finally relinquishing even the will to live. In every case the brain had been literally eaten alive.

Following his hunch, Gajdusek inoculated chimps with tissue taken from CJD victims and found that after years of incubation the monkeys came down with kuru. Obviously CJD and kuru were caused by the same villian, Agent X. Kuru, Gajdusek hypothesized, might have begun when the Fores ate a relative who had spontaneously developed CJD. More important, Gajdusek realized that Agent X was probably at the root of other debilitating disorders of the central nervous system — Parkinson's disease, for example, or Pick's disease, and even Huntington's chorea.

When Gajdusek won the Nobel Prize, in 1976, for his work, he used his prize money to help educate fore youngsters. Relatively little was known about Agent X at the time. The shadowy substance had eluded all scientists' efforts to catch a glimpse of it under electron microscopes, to define its chemical structure, or to explain how it could wreak such havoc. Total knowledge was limited to a few starting facts:

• Agent X caused scrapie, TME, kuru, and CJD.

• Agent X had a slower incubation period than any microorganism known to science.

• Unlike bacteria, viruses, and even tumors, Agent X did not spark the body's immune system into action. It caused no fever, no interferon production, and no identifiable antibodies; only —

eventually—death.

For years the investigation of Agent X was drastically limited by the enormous time that it took to do a single experiment. Marsh studied Agent X by injecting lab animals with scrapie, then watching for results. For each experiment he had to obtain diseased tissue, "brew" an extract of Agent X, and then inject it into a variety of animals. The animals were observed as they slowly incubated the substance—for up to three years. Then, and only then, could they be killed and their tissues be examined for evidence of disease. Because it sometimes took as long as five years to get a single result, it's small wonder that Marsh is eager to abandon his approach in favor of the newer "biochemical techniques" developed by such scientists as Stanley Prusiner, of the University of California at San Francisco.

Prusiner, thirty-nine, is roundish and mild-mannered, a bit like a complacent carpet salesman. He was first fired with curiosity over the mysteries of Agent X while he worked as a medical resident in San Francisco. There his case load included a patient with CJD. So amazed was Prusiner by the woman's rapid neurological debilitation that he stayed in California to track down the substance that was making her ill. Among the most brilliant and energetic newcomers in search of Agent X—he frequently puts in seven days a week at his lab—he assembled a team of ten researchers from such diverse fields as neurochemistry, cell biology, enzymology, and immunology, "to have an expert on hand, no matter what direction our research might lead us in."

At the outset Prusiner was disturbed because no one had yet isolated a pure sample of Agent X. Without such a sample, he knew, it would be virtually impossible to learn much more about the deadly particle. So he set out to isolate the agent, hoping to produce an uncontaminated sample that could be analyzed — and eventually destroyed.

To make large batches of the agent for his first experiments, Prusiner injected mice with brain material from sheep that had scrapie. When the mice died, Prusiner removed their brains and ground them into a pasty liquid.

Prusiner reckoned that out of the entire paste sample, only 1 particle in 1 million was Agent X. To separate that minute quantity from the mass of brain-cell material, he put the paste in a centrifuge and spun it at successively greater speeds. When the centrigue whirled slowly, the heaviest particles spun out of the paste; when it whirled quickly, lighter particles flew away. Prusiner learned that Agent X was a middleweight particle, removed when the centrifuge turned at 50,000 revolutions per minute. By spinning batches of his paste at just that speed, he was able to produce the most concentrated solution of Agent X ever.

But while this sample was stronger than before, Prusiner knew that to produce pure X, he would have to remove many other contaminants. So he subjected the purified paste to hundreds of chemicals, boiled it, and even bombarded it with radiation. In this way he gathered enough information to remove one contaminant after the next: After each procedure, he simply injected the resulting solution into healthy mice. If contaminants were removed and the solution was purified, mice exposed to a more powerful dose of Agent X would become sick more rapidly with less inoculant than before.

Each time a method worked, Prusiner would use it to make batches of a new, more refined solution. The purification went rapidly because Prusiner used a method that enabled him to measure the strength of the agent in a fraction of the time taken by other researchers. Each time he removed a contaminant, he learned something new about the chemical and the physical properties of the agent.

The remarkable outcome is that he and his colleague Frank Masiarz have made batches of Agent X that are 1,000 times as powerful as any found in nature. This lethal Super X has allowed Prusiner to go further than anyone in characterizing slow virus. For instance, he has established that it contains protein, though it does not seem to coat the organism, as it does in viruses. He's also established that if the protein is removed, Agent X loses its infectivity. Once the nature of the protein is determined, physicians will be able to test for infection efficiently. This is a prerequisite for any form of treatment.

Prusiner has also documented that the agent is hydrophobic, that is, that it dislikes watery materials and feels most at home around fatty substances, such as membranes. It also means that Agent X particles probably gather together in well-organized clumps for mutual protection against water.

When challenged, Prusiner recently learned, Agent X particles are defended by a coating of membranelike fat from the body of the stricken person or animal. Thus hidden, they are enormously difficult to identify or destroy.

Prusiner and others are now trying to find out whether Agent X contains nucleic acid, such as DNA. In every form of life discovered on Earth until now, it's been nucleic acid that controlled the transmission of genetic information from one organism to the next. All living cells discovered so far—healthy human cells, bacteria, viruses, tumors—require nucleic acid to reproduce.

Because Agent X does replicate, something must be supervising the process. But so far Prusiner's intensive search for nucleic acid has proved fruitless. And that's the most fascinating part of all. If nobody finds nucleic acid, we may have to revise all previous concepts of how genetic information is passed along. Someday soon one of these hypotheses may be proved true:

• Nucleic acid, such as DNA, is not needed to sustain life in spite of what scientists have thought. If Agent X can transmit genetic information *without* nucleic acid, it will force the scientists back to the drawing board for a new explanation of reproduction.

• Agent X replicates with the aid of nucleic acid from the cells of the organism it has invaded. Thus, it works like a biological switch, turning on systems that cause the body to produce lethal chemicals.

• A tiny bit of nucleic acid may yet be found in Agent X. If it is, it would probably contain one fourth as much information as the smallest virus. That would create a dilemma: Agent X is enormously sophisticated, and its many "behavior patterns" suggest the presence of a large mass of nucleic acid.

• We may never find one answer. Instead, Agent X might be mutating constantly, always one step ahead of body defenses — and researchers. If it has the ability, as well, to repair itself quickly, it may be vulnerable to radiation and life-destroying chemicals; it may only appear to be invulnerable. This might explain why it can lie dormant for so many years, and then cannibalize the brain in just a few months.

These hypotheses have added new excitement to Agent X research. In its last heyday, the drama of a cannibal disease brought new people and new money into the field. This is about to happen again: Scientists struggling to comprehend this bizarre form of life are sure to shake things up, casting serious doubt on some of molecular biology's iron tenets and obliterating others. In the process they could gain enough insight to cure diseases that have plagued man for centuries.

Prusiner recently jet-hopped to three conferences in less than a week. "When I used to run around the world giving papers, my fellow scientists wanted to know what I was wasting my time for," he says. "But this trip was different. Wherever I went, people kept saying to me, 'Boy, Stan, are you lucky you got in when you did!"

FOREVER WAR

By William K. Stuckey

Guillemin and Schally 'laid the foundations for the newest and perhaps most important branch of endocrinology—the study of the hormones produced by the brain itself.' "
— *Science,* April 21, 1978

"Why should I share my data or materials with Guillemin? Does the U.S. share its newest missiles with Russia? There were years of vicious, almost hysterical competition."
— Dr. Andrew Schally, May 2, 1978

"It's been months since Guillemin and Schally won the Nobel Prize, but their fight still goes on. Guillemin just refused to appear on the same stage with Schally at a Stockholm scientific meeting."
— Dr. Samuel McCann, June 2, 1978

"You know the story. Nice guys finish last."
— Dr. Karl Folkers, November 1977

The careers of the cowinners of the 1977 Nobel Prize in Physiology/Medicine, Andrew Schally of Poland and Roger Guillemin of France, have been models of persistence, brilliant intuition, and efficient management—plus fear, jealousy, and character assassination. If their 21-year struggle against their competitors and each other is a general reflection of scientific life, then send your kid to art school. Science is for piranhas.

But while it was sheer hell for the researchers, the Schally-Guillemin quest promises to do as much for the rest of us as the combined discoveries of penicillin, insulin, psychotropic drugs, the Pill, and Spanish fly did. Their still-controversial deciphering of the chemical structures of several hypothalamic hormones may eventually lead to the production of drugs that will control appetite and obesity, prevent blindness and diabetes, control breast and prostrate cancer, improve memory and learning, limit mental instability and increase concentration, and eliminate a large range of human freakishness, including dwarfism.

Perhaps even more dramatic, the Schally-Guillemin accomplishment may allow us to prevent inadvertent baby making on the one hand, and on the other, transform us all into sex objects beyond our most fevered dreams. Yes, the 1977 Nobel Prize research may result in the first effective over-the-counter aphrodisiac, perhaps in the form of a nasal spray. We'll talk more about the future benefits of hormone research later on. But first, a look at the bloodshed . . .

It is extremely rare for scientists to air their dirty linen, and it is difficult to convince them that it is beneficial to do so. For example, an otherwise respected Nobel laureate told me in 1975 that because he disagreed with the mainstream precepts of his science (and with the mainstream leader), he was having difficulty getting research grants, publishing his scientific papers, and obtaining jobs for his students. Yet when I suggested that he provide the names and dates and go public, he was "appalled" at such an idea. The journalistic principal of cure through exposure a la Watergate is an alien one to research and its international symbols, the Swedish judges who award the Nobel Prize. Consequently, we hear essentially the same lament from a losing Schally-Guillemin competitor:

"Look, I can't say too much," he says, pleading for anonymity. "I could still get hurt professionally by . . . well, look, let's skip it. This field is very competitive, with a lot of cutthroat competition. I won't make specific charges, but I know that some of my competitors pulled dirty tricks on me. Schally makes a lot of comments. Guillemin is a very egocentric guy. Schally is aggressive, hard-driving, a cutthroat competitor, but I understand him. Guillemin is harder to understand . . . smoother . . . more cultured."

The unusual thing about the Schally-Guillemin conflict is that Andrew Schally himself has become the whistle blower. He is the first researcher since DNA pioneer James B. Watson (author of *The Double Helix*) to remind us that science not only soars on golden wings but occasionally skids on dog doo.

TALLEYRAND VS. THE PETTY POLE

Science fiction novelist Joe Haldeman might describe the Schally-Guillemin struggle with one of his titles, *The Forever War,* and it is one that Schally sees himself losing in public relations terms. Recently, he sat in his lab at the U.S. Veterans Hospital in New Orleans and waved the latest copy of *Science* magazine at me:

"Always always always," said Schally, who tends to speak in threes. "They are *always* describing Guillemin as urbane and sophisticated, while I am made out to look like a warmonger. *Science* has not treated me fairly."

He referred to an unusual three-part series by Nicholas Wade in the journal of the American Association for the Advancement of Science (April 21 — May 5, 1978). Wade had made a Herculean effort to untangle the complex and heavily disputed chronicle of Schally and Guillemin, but Guillemin seemed to win on points, emerging as Talleyrand, Voltaire, and the Prince of Modesty while Schally emerged as the petty Pole.

The third-party quotes about Guillemin were along the "urbane Frenchman" line; Schally was dismissed as "a Slav in many ways, very excitable." Schally breaks the protocol of the Swedish Nobel Prize judges by admitting that there indeed was a "race" and that yes, it *was* for the Nobel Prize. The Swedes like to think of scientists as truth-seeking Buddhas who would never dream of racing, lobbying, blabbing, or throat cutting for something so intangible as a mere human prize. The Guillemin who appeared in *Science* was made to look like Buddha. *What* race? he asked. *What* prize? Oh yes, his research "required constancy, consistency, and increasing knowhow, but really, there was nothing conceptually revolutionary in this field that made me think a Nobel Prize had to be awarded for it."

There is little doubt as to which of the two is the most personally impressive. Schally has dry, long, and stringy hair combed over bald spots and a voice that often elevates to an incredible, high-pitched whine. Guillemin is bald, with intellectually thin lips, has a trim frame often dressed in something muted and continental (whereas Schally sported emerald-green trousers and scuffy black shoes the day I met him), and owlish eyes reflecting a personal and flattering interest in every inanity a visitor might express. The French-born Guillemin can display noblesse plus oblige. Even his research setting—the austere and elegant castle of the Salk Institute of Biological Studies in La Jolla, California, with majestic views of the Pacific's great whale migration lanes and of cliff-top launching pads for butterflylike hang gliders—far outshines Schally's—a lab that is just down the street from the screaming madhouse of New Orleans's Charity Hospital and with a view of the Superdome.

Schally leads his scientific staff like a combat sergeant. In pursuit of the elusive hypothalamic hormones, he shared the messy job of helping grind up one million pig brains—personally mashing the bean-liked hypothalami with mortar and pestle. Guillemin delegated his own osterizing operation—liquefying six million sheep brains (Schally chose pigs in part because Guillemin had selected sheep)—to a member of his large staff.

I first contacted Schally in November 1977, a few weeks after he had won his share of the Nobel. Ironically, Schally had once worked in the same lab with Guillemin—at Houston's Baylor Medical College, from 1957 to 1962—and I asked how things had been. (I had no knowledge at the time of a blood feud).

"The atmosphere was unbearable. I wouldn't be suppressed and dominated by him any longer," Schally recalled as his voice rose. "I had gone to work for him at Baylor with the understanding that we would be fifty-fifty partners, sharing the credit with each other. He doesn't share credit with anyone. I would not be one of his slaves."

Guillemin, however, took an entirely different and indirect approach when he discussed the Baylor days. Very little was said about Schally at all, except that "he was my student." For fuller information, Guillemin suggested that I speak with venerable Baylor physiologist (and the man who gave Guillemin his first American research post), Hebbel Hoff. Here are selected quotes from Dr. Hoff as to those discrete five years:

• "There was no doubt from the very beginning that the solution of the hypothalamic hormone problem was a problem of Nobel level. Roger was just so clearly in advance in his ideas and technique that nobody ever caught up. Of course, Schally did a great piece of work for Roger, but having him share the Prize with Roger? That's a little bad."

• "I do not think Schally developed any of the basic ideas."

• "When some people are around people of greatness, some people would like to prove to the world that they are just as good."

• In answer to Schally's comment that the atmosphere in Guillemin's Baylor lab was unbearable: "If you considered how long most of Roger's other assistants stayed with him, you would conclude that the laboratory atmosphere was acceptable to most people. But Schally was simply burning to be independent. To that kind of a guy, the atmosphere in anybody else's lab would be unbearable."

• "You have to understand that Schally's father was a general with the Polish government-in-exile during World War II. There is nobody more patriotic than a patriotic Pole. Andrew has transformed that emotion into a search for *la gloire*; you know, winning the Prize. Roger had a little of that tendency. Schally had a lot of it."

If *Science*'s Wade had talked to Hoff, perhaps he would have developed a different view of Guillemin's tactics. (In fairness, however, even some of Schally's coworkers also made extremely harsh indictments of Guillemin—concentrating on his apparently turbulent research career in France—that are too libelous to repeat here.)

And perhaps another view "in fairness" to Roger Guillemin: The man has a postive talent for finding research funds, a talent that induces jealousy in his less fortunate colleagues.

"In the early 1970s," said one competitor (not Schally), "Guillemin came up with several million dollars in grants from the Aid for International Development program. The rest of us didn't even know the money was *there.*"

There is some speculation that the sharpened-elbow race for the Prize also hurt Guillemin and Schally in Swedish eyes. A full half of the $150,000-plus Prize went to Dr. Rosalyn Yalow, of the Veterans Administration Hospital in the Bronx, for developing the radioactive-tracer assay techniques that permitted Guillemin and Schally to pinpoint the two-dimensional chemical structures of the first three hypothalamic hormones. Dr. Yalow's achievements apparently have aroused no ire. The Frenchman and the Pole had to be content with a quarter-slice each.

But Schally is forever. Not only does he continue to call a Guillemin a Guillemin, but he implies that his future work will be of such quality that an unprecedented second medical Nobel is not out of the question. It is presumed that he would prefer not to share it with Roger Guillemin.

CHILDREN IN NAZILAND

Twenty-one years of hand-to-hand combat being unusual, one looks at the early backgrounds for some answers. And the reasons for both Guillemin's and Schally's toughness may be found there. Guillemin spent his teens living in Nazi-occupied France, while the slightly younger Schally underwent a similar ordeal in Poland before he and his parents escaped to Scotland (where life was only slightly better during the great "British Austerity" period following the war). The sole anecdotes that survive this period of Guillemin's life are that he was wounded — by an artillery shell from invading Americans — and that he was connected with a country hospital that was actually a front for the French Resistance.

Perhaps the Guillemin manner was also honed in the stifling formalities of the French university (he received his M.D. from his hometown University of Dijon and joined the medical faculty at Lyons during the early postwar period). Later, during his tenure at Baylor in the 1950s and '60s, he accepted a joint appointment with the College de France, an arrangement that to the delight of the Schally forces apparently did not work out. Guillemin-supporter Hoff provides these details:

"Roger just ran into the total failure of the French system. There was inadequate interest in or support for his research. Their system is so terribly antique. There are too many old professors appointed for life and no breathing room for the younger people. And Roger is certainly not the first Nobel-level scientist that the French boo-booed on. André Cournand had tried in vain to get a job in France but finally had to settle for Columbia University — where his research won him the Prize (for heart catheterization) in 1956."

Schally went into chemistry in England, working for a while in the Laureate-rich atmosphere of London's National Institute for Medical Research. He describes this period as a pleasant one, and one that gave him a character dissimilar to that of his great competitor.

"Well, you see, we have different characters," Schally analyzed. "I was brought up in England, and I'm quite proud of it. We never do something, never do anything behind someone's back. We are very ethical. I am hard, but very ethical. Yes yes yes. Guillemin believes, you know, diplomacy, Talleyrand, at which the French excel, very political. If I don't like something, I'll just say so."

Question: Are you saying that Guillemin is the type to do things behind people's back?

"I would never do that," replied Schally.

Question: But are you saying *he* would?

"I'm not saying that. We are different types. I like sports, he hates sports, my health has always been excellent, his is bad . . . "

Question: How did you get along with him in Stockholm at the Prize ceremonies?

"Oh, Guillemin was extremely proper, extremely friendly, he was even cordial. I didn't feel like being cordial, but he was."

Does it never end? But wait, there *is* some science in this narrative.

FOG IN THE LABS
"Up in my head,
Just over my tongue,
A little thing from my brain is hung.
To make it work there are factors new
That tell it when and how much to pitu."
— Professor Murray Saffran.

Science, April 21, 1978

Andrew Schally left England for Montreal's
McGill University in 1952, where for the next five
years he copublished papers with Professor Saffran. Their research task was a radical one in hormone circles. Several other scientists, including
the late Geoffrey Harris of Oxford, who probably would have shared the 1977 Prize with Schally
et al if he had not broken a Prize-eligibility rule
by doggerel description of the "little thing from
my brain," the pituitary, was *not* the body's master gland that regulated the most important hormonal traffic. The clues were that another organ,
the hypothalamus, actually told the pituitary
what to do by squirting out "hormone releasing"
factors through a hypothalamic-pituitary blood
vessel network.

The problem had the richest of Nobel Prize elements. As a classical problem, it would be a rare
coup to disprove the decades-old pituitary "master gland" theory by the "discovery"—the key
Nobel buzzword, first articulated in the 1896 will
of Alfred Nobel himself—that the hypothalamus
held the true power over sex, growth, response of
the body to physical stress (cold, heat, infection,
etc.), and other intriguing functions. And isolating and unscrambling the chemical structure of
releasing factors would meet Alfred Nobel's crite-
rion of being of "benefit to mankind"—since the
chemistry hopefully could be modified, producing drugs that could diagnose or right hormonal
wrongs in a much quicker, cheaper, and more effective way than tampering with the delicate pituitary itself. According to Saffran, he and Schally
saw the Nobel significance in hypothalamic hormones immediately, with Schally beginning the

search for the extremely elusive factors as early as 1954.

A classic mystery suggested that the pituitary master-control theory was wrong. The mystery is the young girl, a virgin, who under the stress of leaving home for the first time (or other nonsexual stresses), misses her period for six months or so. If the prevailing pituitary theory was correct, the situation would be impossible, since the theory states that the pituitary pumps key sex hormones into the bloodstream with unfailing accuracy and independently of emotion. Perhaps, then, the hypothalamus, which presumably does react to outside "stressful" information such as visual images and emotions, was responsible for the girl's irregularity. And if this is true for sex, why not for other hormonally controlled functions? The hypothalamus and its mysterious releasing factors added a weird, mind-over-matter quality to classical anatomy.

Roger Guillemin also had become interested in stress and hormonal function, having also moved to Canada wor work under the University of Montreal's Hans Selye, a Nobel-connected nabob if ever there was one and an authority on stress. He writes (in Plenum Publishing's *Pioneers of Neuroendocrinology,* 1978) that he came to the hypothalamic-control idea independently, then heard of "Saffran's work" (no mention at all of Schally, who nevertheless was a coauthor of the first research papers) and wrote him for information.

Guillemin then shifted his research base to Houston. Young Schally, hearing that the Texas Frenchman shared mutual research interest, wrote from Montreal, asking to work in Guillemin's Houston lab. Guillemin notes icily (in *Pi-*

oneers that Professor Saffran, Schally's overseer, gave Schally a "guarded" recommendation. But Guillemin hired Schally anyway, and Schally began the first of his five "unbearable" years before bolting to New Orleans to head his own VA-sponsored research drive.

The problem is that the rest of the world of endocrinology—except for Dallas's Dr. Samuel McDonald McCann and a handful of other hearty since-the-1950s pioneers—thought Guillemin and Schally were totally wrong. Moreover, they began to suspect over the years that the two spent more time going for each other's jugular (at acridly atmosphered scientific meetings and in the pages of journals) than trying to solve they hypothalamic problem. Guillemin and Schally had wasted years chasing the structure of the wrong releasing factor (corticotropin releasing factor, or CRF). Schally says that he and Saffran believed they were presenting, with CRF, the "first direct proof of the existence of hypothalamic hormones," but that the insubstantial nature of the chemical itself, plus inadequate analyzing tools, prevented their determining its exact chemical structure.

Both Guillemin and Schally, each hot on the other's heels, shifted to the structure of a less problematic releasing factor, thyroid releasing hormone (TRH). Then, at an unusual meeting in Tucson in 1969—called by the National Institute of Health (NIH) backers of the competing teams of Guillemin and Schally to determine if the Pole and the Frenchman were really going to accomplish anything—Guillemin pulled a dazzler.

Guillemin announced that he had come up with a TRH sample pure enough (that is, separated from the extraneous head tissues of all those sheep brains) to at last begin work on its structure. The NIH, which had been prepared to suspend the research funds for both scientists, relented and stopped laughing.

The problem for Guillemin was that Schally himself had TRH in "pure form" and had identified its three-amino-acid sequence *three years before* but believed then that he was wrong.

The nature of the burdens on the Swedish Prize judges, who must determine who did what first, begins to be perceived.

Then, along came Karl Folkers of the University of Texas at Austin to roil the waters even more. Folkers, a crack chemist, was asked by Schally to help him work out the final TRH structure. Folkers did—"at least several weeks before Guillemin's team did." Today, Guillemin will not speak of Folkers. When I asked Guillemin to comment on the Folkers work, he replied: "I wish no comment on that person. No, change that and say, I wish no comment on that colleague."

Schally also downplays Folker's work on the stuctural problem. Ironically, it is not Schally or Guillemin—but Karl Folkers—who holds the patent on TRH structure.

A note on all that animal mush: Guillemin's most brilliant research stroke in pursuing the extremely potent, small, and hard-to-isolate releasing factors was in the sheer volume of sheep brains he decided had to be processed for hypothalamic truths. Six million brains, which he bought from packing houses at 40 cents apiece (a total of $2.4 million), only hints at the total amount of public and private funds spent by the two in their 21-year search. Schally kept abreast with his one million pig brains—donated free by the Oscar Mayer weenie people. Dr. McCann, the pride of the physiology at Dallas's University of Texas Health Sciences Center, speculates that he probably did not survive in the Nobel sweep-stakes because he simply did not want to convert his lab into an industrial brain-blending facility.

"After we processed about 75,000 brains, I said that was enough," McCann recalled. "It is not very interesting work, and the funding wasn't all that good either. I was more interested in the physiology of how the hypothalamus actually controls the pituitary, if it does, than in solving a mundane chemical structure problem.

Wait a minute. *If* it does?

The score card on the three structures mapped to date, which was enough to convince the Swedes of the research's Nobel quality, is as follows:

Thyroid releasing hormone. Guillemin claims a win: Schally concedes a draw — although co-workers say they had it in pure form years before Guillemin; but Karl Folkers holds the patent. (Analysis: Try the polygraph.)

Luteinizing Hormone Releasing Hormone (LHRH, which directs the pituitary in timing ov-ulation and sexual behavior). Schally apparently scored a clean sweep here in structural decipher-ing, although the Texan, McCann, is given credit for first isolating it in hypothalamic extracts.

Somatostatin (which, among other things, in-hibits the action of growth hormones and affects insulin production in diabetics) is also claimed by Guillemin. But add this dissenting note from Mc-Cann: 'We published four articles on somatos-tatin before Guillemin did. Meanwhile, he was badmouthing the existence of somatostatin and claimed that our results could not be duplicated in his lab. Baloney."

One almost feels a surge of sympathy for the Swedish truth seekers and Prize finders, particularly after the comments of another Dallas hypothalamic worker, Dr. John Porter:

"No one yet knows exactly how the hypothalamus drives the pituitary, or *if* it does," said Dr. Porter. "We are now finding some of these substances, like somatostatin, all over the brain and elsewhere in the body, not just in the hypothalamus. All we know is that something goes into the pituitary and something goes out. It's a typical black box explanation: here's what happens, but we don't know why. The Prize to Guillemin and Schally, I believe, was strictly for a technological feat. They got the two-dimensional structure of the releasing factors. Fine. That tells us how to modify it and make useful pharmaceuticals. But we still don't know the three-dimensional structure. Look at the Nobel Prize for Watson-Crick's model of DNA. That was three-dimensional . . . *conceptual*. The structure suggests exactly how genetic material reproduces itself. All we know about releasing factors is what amino acid follows what other amino acid. No conceptual breakthroughs there. Again, though, we gained a useful new class of therapeutic agents."

One is reminded here of Guillemin's own comment in *Science* about there being nothing "conceptually revolutionary" about the releasing-factor field.

Where does that leave the Swedes and Andrew Schally? It leaves the Swedes in Stockholm and Andrew Schally still generally happy as a clam and thinking about sex in a mind-over-matter way.

LOVE, SCIENCE & OTHER TALES

"I'm on top now," said a greatly relaxed Schally. "I got here without dirty tricks. No no no. Nothing of the sort. It has never been my way to play tricks. I went to Stockholm in 1973, and sources on the Nobel Committee at the very highest level told me that LHRH [the sex hormone-releasing factor] was definitely my victory scientifically. The structures of only three releasing factors have been solved so far. With the Prize, I will not become a politician but will continue my original interests, trying to solve the other structures. We were the first to demonstrate the activity of the *antagonistic analogues* [chemical modifications that inhibit sex hormone action] in LHRH, so we are placing heavy emphasis on new methods of birth control. Without side effects: Probably still to be taken daily, but perhaps by nasal spray. At the same time, we are developing clinically *stimulatory analogues* [which enhance sex hormone production] to sexually stimulate men and women, to overcome psychogenic impotence."

Stimulate? Didn't Wade say in *Science* something about LHRH studies that might produce true aphrodisiacs? Is he working on aphrodisiacs? Is that too strong a word?

"Uh . . . well, yes and no," Andrew Schally replies. "I'm not saying I have them. I am just saying that psychiatrist and clinicians should explore the potentials of analogues."

Any chance of a mass-produced aphrodisiac ever hitting the stores?

"(Laughs). Certainly. But not every man might respond to it. We need many more double-blind studies. There is also evidence that LHRH is a good antidepressant, so that might explain a possible aphrodisiac effect. The effect has definitely been shown in animals. Published by others, not me. It could be used to increase libido, or something like that."

Come on, won't it work on women too?

"I could tell you many stories over a glass of wine, but without the double-blind studies, they could not be accepted. I still don't want to talk about it. But if this [aphrodisiac] effect is found, it wouldn't at all surprise me."

Would it be the kind of thing you might slip into someone's drink?

"Well . . . like Spanish fly? You could do that with Spanish fly too. But that is harmful. You would destroy the liver and kidneys and the genito-urinary tract. No, you couldn't take a new aphrodisiac orally. You would inject it or use a nasal spray."

(Since winning the Prize, Schally has indulged himself in one public macho joke. To the press in New Orleans he mentioned that his new wife, from Brazil, was also an endocrinologist who "did beautiful work with my hormones.")

But Schally has other interests.

"I also want to prepare analogues of somatostatin, not only for control of ulcers but for prevention of blindness that occurs with several types of diabetes. My research is planned at least fifteen or twenty years in advance. Later, we will take on central [brain] control of the appetite and obesity. I have already published a few theories about hypothalamic control of obesity. I also want to work on some aspects of cancer, principally breast and prostate, which may respond to some analogues of the releasing factors. I also want to see how some of these factors might control general behavior — sex, learning, and so on. We have indications. Perhaps we will find out how to improve the memory. Yes yes. Of course I do not intend to share any of this with Guillemin. Did Watson and Crick share their findings with Linus Pauling?"

CONTAMINATED SCIENCE

By Owen Davies

Nightmares of lost years, grants, and reputations are galloping through the heads of researchers these days, thanks to a new outbreak of "defectitis." In this dread affliction, competent scientists suddenly lose control over their work and are no longer able to make sense of their experiments. Carefully designed studies collapse into terminal confusion or, worse, yield misinformation that can mislead other scientists for years.

The cause is defective research materials: mongrel mice sold as genetically pure varieties, contaminated or mislabeled cell cultures, and similar snares for the unwary. Many conclusions of medical research are meaningless unless the scientists know precisely the genetic makeup of their research subjects. Studies involving immunology are particularly vulnerable, notably cancer and organ-transplantation research.

No one knows how often fatal flaws appear,

but it seems certain that they are far more common than most scientists acknowledge. Dr. Walter Nelson-Rees, who recently retired from the University of California's Naval Biosciences Research Laboratory, in Oakland, has spent more than a decade tracking down faulty tissue cultures. Last year he compiled a list of contaminated cultures that he and others had uncovered; 130 had been reported. Most had been taken over by HeLa cells, a common and rapidly growing line of cancer cells. Others had been misidentified: Mouse cells were labeled as guinea-pig cells; "frog cells" were a mix of box-turtle and minnow cells; and supposedly human tissues had come from rats, mice, hamsters, and monkeys.

One such mishap destroyed five years of research into Hodgkin's disease—a cancer of the lymph nodes, spleen, and liver—and ended the career of the scientists responsible for it. In the mid-Seventies Dr. John Long, who was at Massachusetts General Hospital, in Boston, announced that he had managed to grow four cultures of cells taken from Hodgkin's patients. This was a goal that had eluded researchers for many years. The triumph made Dr. Long's reputation and seemed to give Hodgkin's specialists an important new tool.

Then one of Long's experiments produced findings so odd that a leading scientific journal rejected his report just when he needed a new grant to continue his work. Sure that his cell cultures were trustworthy and yet unable to explain his results, Long succumbed to the pressure. He forged data that won the support he required.

When the deception was discovered late in 1979, Long was allowed to resign from the hospital on the condition that he never return to research. Today he works as a hospital pathologist in the Midwest.

Long's departure did not end the matter, however, for behind him he had left a mystery far more important than his fraud: Were his cultures really cells obtained from Hodgkin's patients? If not, some fundamental insights into the disease would have to be rethought.

Dr. Nancy Harris, who had worked with Long on a prestigious two-year fellowship from the National Institutes of Health, was assigned to find out. It took her six months. The breakthrough came when Dr. Nelson-Rees managed to confirm her suspicion: Not only were they not Hodgkin's-cell cultures, but three of them were not even cultures of human cells. Another consultant soon identified them as belonging to a Colombian brown-footed owl monkey. Long had contaminated his original cultures with cells from another experiment, and the hardy simian cells had replaced the human ones.

In all, it was a costly error. Long's career was lost; so was a bit more than $300,000 in research funds spent before his deception came to light. And then there was the five-year period in which his error may have misled countless other investigators.

Dr. Harris's future in research may also have been jeopardized. "I had only those two years in which to carry out research without clinical duties," she says. "Since then I have limited myself to working with patients. I have not applied for any funding. I spent two full years and produced no original results. It's difficult to justify any further investment in my research after that."

Errors involving whole animals are less frequent, but when they do occur, they can be disastrous. In one recent incident Dr. Brenda Kahan, of the University of Wisconsin, was studying chimeric mice, animals whose bodies contain cells derived from the fertilized egg as well as foreign cells injected into the growing embryo. The choice of the mice used, a variety called BALB/c, was crucial to the study.

But when Dr. Kahan grew her chimeras and tested their cells, she found that the parent mice could not have been BALB/c. She and Dr. Robert Auerback eventually traced the error to Charles River Breeding Laboratories. For nearly a year the firm had been selling hybrid mice, identifying these animals as purebred BALB/c. Apparently one of the breeding animals had escaped and was put back into a wrong cage.

To medical scientists, the discovery is chilling. Charles River is the world's largest supplier of lab animals: BALB/c is one of its most often used varieties. "The seriousness of our findings cannot be overemphasized," Drs. Kahan and Auerbach state. Charles River's mistake cost them nearly a year of work and up to $100,000 in wasted research funds. And because the BALB/c is so common, hundreds of other investigators may have suffered the same misfortune. It will be several years before the full extent of the calamity is known.

"This has really put a scare into people," says Dr. Harold Hoffman, who directs the program in genetic quality control for the National Institutes of Health. "Studies in immunology and toxicology are the ones most at risk. It can cost a million dollars to set up your lab to test the safety of a single drug, and there are about fifty-five drugs now waiting to be tested. This kind of error could ruin that research."

It is possible to guard against defective research materials, but it is far from easy. Genetic testing of tissue cultures is painstaking and specialized work, which few laboratories can afford to perform routinely. Several consulting laboratories plan soon to offer such quality-control services, but there is much more work to be done than they can hope to accomplish.

Dr. Hoffman's laboratory works full time to guard the genetic purity of the 20 strains of lab animals produced there. In the past five years six potentially damaging problems have been brought to light, including two natural mutations. But Hoffman's is the only program of its kind in this country.

Drs. Kenneth Pennline and Hinrick Bitter-Suerman, of George Washington University, in St. Louis, recently solved such a problem—after losing more than a year's work on transplant immunology because a major animal supplier in England had sent them the wrong mice. "Eventually we bought two hundred mice, tested all of them, and used only the ones that we knew were right," Dr. Pennline reports. "There were thirty-seven of them."

At best, it's a poor solution. "That's horrible to contemplate," Dr. Kahan declares. "Not many people can do that kind of check before an experiment."

Pennline agrees. "Dr. Bitter-Suerman is working to get legislation that would force animal suppliers to use better quality control," he reports. "It should not be necessary to check up on them."

But until such legislation is enacted, the penalty for not checking can be even worse than the inconvenience of doing so. "We were getting into a very productive period in our work," Pennline recalls. "It shut down as if a ton of bricks had fallen on it. With the field as competitive as it is, and grant money becoming increasingly scarce, you just can't afford to lose a year.

"That isn't the worst of it," he adds. "When your experiments fail and you can't figure out why, you begin to lose your enthusiasm. You slack off. Your colleagues know you're not doing your best anymore, and it damages your relationship with them. That's the part that really hurts."

PART EIGHT:
BIOETHICS

SO THAT OTHERS MAY LIVE

By Dava Sobel

Somebody always has to be the guinea pig, because everything that's ever learned about medicine gets tested, sooner or later, on a human subject. Many of those subjects have been scientists themselves, infecting their own bodies with mystery diseases or instructing that certain surgical procedures be performed on them first. Many more have been patients whose doctors have "experimented" during therapy, trying several different paths toward a cure. And an untold number of humans have been the willing or unwitting subjects of experiments performed not for their benefit but in the interest of science.

Human experimentation is as fixed an element of research as theories or test tubes are. Yet the words make the skin crawl and conjure up visions of Nazi-doctor horrors and the brutal exploitation of prisoners, poor people, and hospital patients. Knowledge that such things can and do happen has gradually made suspect, for a variety of ethical reasons, all kinds of human investigations — from test-tube fertilization to questionnaires on sex. Today new regulations have produced safeguards that have actually stopped certain studies altogether, put limits on many others, and frozen the rest in landfills of red tape. We can't help wondering how all this will affect the future course of medical discovery.

Consider the frustrations of Dr. Pierre Soupart, a professor of obstetrics and gynecology at Vanderbilt University, in Nashville, Tennessee. Soupart's goal is to study what he calls "the unknown realm of the first six days of pregnancy" — research that involves test-tube fertilization. But he has been unable to obtain a federal grant because, in August 1975, the federal government withdrew funding of all projects involving the fertilization of human eggs in laboratory glassware.

Apparently reeling under the ethical implications of this work, the Department of Health, Education and Welfare (HEW) charged its Ethics Advisory Board with the task of considering the moral issues raised by test-tube fertilization. Unfortunately, the 14 board members were not appointed until February 1978, and they made no recommendations until March of this year, when they deemed Soupart's work ethically acceptable. As of this writing, however, HEW is still collecting public response to the board's decision, and the ban remains in effect. So while Soupart continued to conduct peripheral studies and give lectures, other researchers at private American facilities proceed unhindered. And a baby named Louise Brown was born in England.

Commenting on why his study has met such resistance, Soupart cites the "slippery slope argument," fear that once in vitro fertilization and embryo transfer are proved feasible, a brave new world of test-tube babies and imagined horrors will follow. Soupart's intention is not to produce test-tube babies. He is not even sure he would want to implant one of his laboratory-bench embryos into a woman's body, although the Ethics Advisory Board sees nothing wrong with the idea, provided the sperm and ovum come from a married couple.

"In any kind of human-subjects research," Soupart says, "the only way to determine the validity of the research proposal is by balancing the risks against the potential benefits. You don't get anything for nothing. So you must decide whether the benefits from the new knowledge justify the risks you take to get the knowledge."

And who should make that decision? The scientist who may underplay the risk? Or an ethicist who may underestimate the benefit?

In the usual course of human-subjects research today. the subjects themselves are the ultimate judges: When a scientist applies for money to start a research project, the funding agency asks other scientists to review the idea. If these peers judge the experiment scientifically unnecessary or excessively risky, they kill it with their disapproval. In addition, the Institutional Review Board (IRB) at a scientists's home institution weighs the risk to human subjects and determines how the subjects will be informed of those risks. Even after getting IRB approval and agency funding, a scientist must still *invite* people to participate as subjects, and they are free to say yes or no.

Imagine Edward Jenner trying to perform his landmark vaccination experiments in this climate. How likely would he have been to get institutional approval of plans to inject eight-year-old Master Phipps with fluid from a milkmaid's cowpox blister? And only two months later to inoculate the same child with smallpox, the most dreaded disease of the day, to test his hoped-for immunity?

Beyond the protection of peer review and informed consent, a willing subject can sign the informed-consent papers, participate, and then decide later that he was not really fully informed. At that point he could sue the investigator for any ill effects he felt he had suffered. Human-subjects research might thus become nearly as fertile a field for legal action as medical malpractice is. And in the social sciences, other ethical problems arise: Even if a subject agrees to answer survey questions about his criminal activities or his sexual preferences, how can we ensure that his answers are kept confidential? If someone gains access to the data files in a computer, what is a scientist's legal or ethical liability?

The problems have grown so tangled and so numerous that a new periodical called *IRB* appeared in March of this year, promising ten issues annually to help practitioners unravel "ethical dilemmas posed by research, regulations governing research, and the decision-making process itself."

The publisher of *IRB* is the Hastings Center, just outside New York City, where staff members make a practice of considering unwieldy questions in biomedical and behavioral research from the right to live to the right to die. When asked how the restrictions on human-subjects research might affect important investigations in the next several years, medical ethics associate Robert Veatch said, "I don't think that any kind of drug- or disease-related studies will be hampered at all. We're convinced that these can be done ethically. But many kinds of social research that we've seen could not be funded in today's climate of ethical review."

UNTOLD VICTIMS

Popular concern for the welfare of human subjects is relatively new. This concern dates from the 1945—46 Nuremberg trials, when the crimes committed in the concentration camps were openly discussed and moral codes for conducting "experiments" were formalized. Before that, all the way back through 4,000 years of records kept by doctor-priests and scientists who experimented on people, researchers had just let their conscience be their guide.

Even after Nuremberg, there was no appreciable change in ethical standards. Many misguided zealots continued to involve human beings in dangerous experiments, with catastrophic results. As recently as 1966 a Harvard University physician had to call public attention to the inexcusable treatment of human subjects right here at home, in America's "leading medical schools, university hospitals, private hospitals, military departments (the army, the navy, and the air force), governmental institutes (the National Institutes of Health). Veterans Administration hospitals, and industry." Writing in the *New England Journal of Medicine* (June 16, 1966), Dr. Henry K. Beecher cataloged example after chilling example:

"Artificial induction of hepatitis was carried out in an institution for mentally defective children," Beecher reported. "The parents gave consent for the intramuscular injection or oral administration of the virus, but nothing is said regarding what was told them concerning the appreciable hazards involved . . . ."

"Live cancer cells were injected into 22 human subjects as part of a study of immunity to cancer. According to a recent review, the subjects [hospitalized patients] were 'merely told they would be receiving "some cells" . . . the word *cancer* was entirely omitted . . . .'

"Twenty-six normal babies less than 48 hours old . . . were exposed to X rays while their bladder was filling and during voiding. Multiple spot films were made to record the presence or absence of ureteral reflux. None was found in this group, and fortunately no infection followed the catheterization. What the results of the extensive x-ray exposure may be, no one can yet say."

Beecher said his point was not to identify or condemn individual researchers or even to document the worst cases he could find. Rather, he was trying to prove how many kinds of "ethical errors" were possible and how these would multiply as funding for medical research grew.

Crying for a way to enforce "responsible" investigation, he suggested that journals refuse to publish results that were unethically obtained. And he implored researchers to "strive" to explain the aim of their experiments, and especially the hazards, to their potential subjects, so these people could either give informed consent or refuse to participate.

The infamous "Tuskegee study" of syphilis, involving hundreds of intentionally untreated cases of the disease, was not even mentioned in Beecher's paper. This experimentation was sponsored by the Venereal Diseases Division of the U.S. Public Health Service. The subjects of this research were 399 black men from Macon County, Alabama, all twenty-five years old or older, who were selected because they had advanced cases of syphilis and had never received any treatment for it. There was also a control group of 201 nonsyphilitic males, also black, and 275 more who had been inadequately treated for syphilis years before. The point of the study was to observe the men and trace the course of the untreated disease so as to understand its "natural history."

In 1932, when the study participants were selected, penicillin was unknown, although mercury had been prescribed for syphilis since medieval times and newer treatments (arsphenamine, introduced in 1910, bismuth compounds, in 1922) were proving to be more effective. Many people with syphilis never sought treatment, yet they sometimes seemed to recover spontaneously, leading a few doctors to believe one might be better off without the dangerous chemicals. Nobody knew for sure, however, and that missing bit of knowledge ostensibly justified the study's objective.

After the first critical report of the Tuskegee activities appeared in *The New York Times* on July 26, 1972, public interest and revulsion gathered so quickly that the study was terminated within four months, and no monograph of the 40 years of data has yet been published.

PRISONERS OF SCIENCE

In America's prisons, men who served as "human experimental material" fared even worse, receiving $1 a day in 1971 to be fed vitamin-deficient diets through stomach tubes until they developed scurvy, to be exposed to cholera or poisonous insecticides, to receive (in 1962) toxic injections to test their pain tolerance, to submit to daily applications of caustic substances on their skin, to be bitten by mosquitoes for ten minutes at a time, or to have pieces of muscle tissue removed from their arms.

When Jessica Mitford wrote her prison expose, *Kind and Usual Punishment*, in 1971, a University of California scientist said to her, "If the researchers really believe these experiments are safe for humans, why do they go to the prisons for subjects? Why don't they try them out in their own laboratories on their own students or other 'free-world' volunteers? Because they know the university would never permit this. And, furthermore, it would never enter their minds to do these things to people they associate with in daily life. They make a clear distinction between people they think of as social equals or colleagues and men behind bars; whom they regard as less than human."

The U.S. government began to phase out medical experiments in federal penitentiaries in 1973, and no new studies have since been started. The last ongoing federal prison project ended in 1977, although there is still some scattered activity in a few state prisons. One of the decisive arguments against the use of prisoners — even when they are fully informed and paid for their services — is that they are in no position to give consent with freedom of choice. ("If a man is in a cell with several other violent men," one philosopher proposed to me, "and you offer him a private hospital room with a TV if he'll participate in an experiment, what do you think he'll say?") Drug companies, which relied on prison populations for testing new compounds, have turned to students and other so-called organized populations, just as Mitford's friend suggested. The more dangerous experiments have apparently been stopped.

As I write this, new evidence of past ethical infractions is emerging in Illinois, where the Cook County public guardian claims that researchers removed the adrenal glands from an unknown number of mental patients at a University of Chicago hospital during the 1950s and 1960s.

Offsetting the painful accounts of human exploitation are the unsung stories of ethically conducted research and the tales of investigators who tried nothing on a human subject before putting themselves to the test first. Dr. Lawrence K. Altman, a medical writer for *The New York Times*, has been collecting case histories for 15 years to write a book about autoexperimentation, which will be published soon by Random House. Chapters will tell of:

• Anton Storck, of Austria, who swallowed hemlock in increasing doses for more than a week, proving in 1760 that the substance could be taken without undue danger for the treatment of cancer, tumors, ulcers, and cataracts;

• William Stark, of England, who at age twenty-nine put himself on a diet of bread and water, variously augmented by sugar, eggs, olive oil, salt, figs, or various meats, to test which foods were "hurtful," which "innocent." He died for his efforts in 1770, before his thirtieth birthday;

• Roscoe R. Spencer, of Hamilton, Montana, who administered to himself the first test on a human being of the Spencer Parker Rocky Mountain spotted fever vaccine in 1924; and

• Werner Forssmann, of Germany, who proved the feasibility of cardiac catheterization in 1929, by maneuvering a 65-centimeter-long "well-oiled ureter catheter" into a vein near his left elbow and on through to his heart, recounting later how "even the rather long trip in our institution from the operating room to the x-ray department, during which I had to climb stairs, traveling on foot with the catheter located in the heart, was not associated with any annoyance."

The federal authorities have no truck with self-experimenters because, clearly, those who subject themselves to their own research at least understand the risks involved. It's everybody else who needs protecting.

How can this be done?

With money. Or, more specifically, with the threat of withholding money.

The government, through HEW, will not fund any research that involves the unethical treatment of human subjects. And if one lone researcher at an enormous university starts an experiment without first getting informed consent from the subjects, the entire institution could lose *all* its support from HEW and the National Institutes of Health (NIH). The government requires every university receiving federal money to police its own scientists and has established laws and guidelines for doing so. Obey, or forfeit all grants; it's that simple.

At large drug companies, where most research is funded by profit, the government exerts a different kind of leverage: All drugs and devices must be approved by the Food and Drug Administration (FDA) before they can be sold. Steps toward approval include animal trials and various tests on human subjects. And if the human experiments don't match the FDA's ethical standards (which approximate those of HEW), the drug will not be approved.

Most human-subjects research is now covered by these safeguards. But, according to Charles MacKay, deputy director of the NIH Office of Protection from Research Risk, no federal law applies to the goings-on in privately funded institutions. Thus, David Rorvik's tale of human cloning — financed in secret by a millionaire who wanted a son exactly like himself — was *legally*, if not scientifically, feasible.

IN DEFENSE OF DECEPTION

The diverse kinds of valuable social research that Robert Veatch says "coulld not be funded in today's climate of ethical review" would probably include Stanley Milgram's "obedience experiments" at Yale in 1960 — 62, where more than 1,000 participants had to be misinformed in order to learn which behavior was the more typical obedience to authority or compassion for a person in pain. Milgram, now a professor of psychology at the City University of New York, described the work himself in his book *Obedience to Authority: An Experimental View* (Harper & Row, 1974).

Milgram writes, "Two people come to a psychology laboratory to take part in a study of memory and learning. One of them is designated a teacher and the other, a learner. The experimenter explains that the study is concerned with the effects of punishment on learning. The learner is conducted into a room, seated in a chair, his arms strapped to prevent excessive movement, and an electrode is attached to his wrist. He is told that he is to learn a list of work pairs; whenever he makes an error, he will receive electric shocks of increasing intensity.

"The real focus of the experiment is on the teacher. After watching the learner being strapped into place, he is taken into the main experimental room and seated before an impressive shock generator. Its main feature is a horizontal line of 30 switches, ranging from 15 volts to 450 volts, in 15-volt increments. There are also verbal designations which range from SLIGHT SHOCK to DANGER—SEVERE SHOCK. The teacher is told that he is to administer the learning test to the learner in the other room. When he responds correctly, the teacher moves on to the next item; when the learner gives an incorrect answer, the teacher is to give him an electric shock. He is to start at the lowest shock level . . . and to increase the level each time the man makes an error. . . .

"The teacher is a genuinely naïve subject who has come to the laboratory to participate in an experiment. The learner, or victim, is an actor who actually receives no shock at all. . . .

"Conflict arises when the man receiving the shock begins to indicate that he is experiencing discomfort. At 75 volts, the learner grunts. At 120 volts, he complains verbally; at 150, he demands to be released from the experiment. His protests continue as the shocks escalate, growing increasingly vehement and emotional. At 285 volts, his response can only be described as an agonized scream.

"Observers of the experiment agree that its gripping quality is somewhat obscured in print. For the subject, the situation is not a game; conflict is intense and obvious . . . . "

Milgram points out that 80 percent of social-psychology research requires staging or technical illusion and that laws against such procedures would greatly interfere with inquiry.

"Of course, you can't withhold information

that affects the person's willingness to participate in the experiment," Milgram said in an interview, "but you must withhold certain information for epistemological reasons. If the subjects of this kind of research were *fully* informed, experiments would become meaningless."

He added, "I think it's much more risky to swallow some unknown chemical than to participate in this kind of study. And there is no evidence whatsoever that when an individual makes a choice in a laboratory situation — even the difficult choices posed by the conformity or obedience experiments — any trauma, injury, or diminution of well-being results."

Yet, Milgram points out, some of the proposed regulations in this area would make it impossible for a trained scientist to conduct market research — "while any person on the street is free to ask questions of anybody." Milgram finds this an absurd possibility, indicating, he thinks, that the degree of regulation may have reached its peak.

But if not, there will have to be new solutions to the problem of pursuing human-subjects research. Might there be a place in some future job market for professional human-subjects-research, where people like Evel Knievel could put their daring to public service? Veatch says no. "A subject actually becomes useless with experience," he explained. "The more you do to him, the less 'normal' he becomes. Either he's had too many drugs in his system, or he's gotten too savvy about research protocol and begins to say what he thinks the investigator wants to hear."

SCARCITY OF MONKEYS

Arthur Caplan, another Hastings Center staffer and a member of Columbia University's institutional review board, says that human research will continue to expand despite tighter government scrutiny.

"There's a monkey shortage," Caplan said, "and a real potential in Western society for concern about animals' rights to increase to the point where it poses a problem for research in general — and people in general — because less animal experimentation will only mean more human experimentation."

The Indian government stopped exporting rhesus monkeys to the United States last year, abruptly ending an annual supply of 12,000 animals for needed testing of vaccines and other drugs. Some South American countries (Brazil, Peru, Colombia) had already embargoed their commercial primate trade when the latest shortage occurred. At regional primate centers around the country, U. S. scientists are trying to breed captive populations of experimental monkeys from existing supplies, but, so far, native production is no match for the missing imports. For most research purposes involving monkeys, other animals simply will not do. And as for skipping the monkey step and proceeding directly to human volunteers, well, no one has suggested that. Yet.

"One of the hard facts of life for the twenty-first-century researchers is that the diseases are tougher than ever," Caplan continued. "Cancer and stroke are much less amenable to miraculous cures than were measles, anthrax, and smallpox. Self-experimentation will play only a minimal role. For, while Walter Reed and his boys had no problem acquiring yellow fever, the future researcher may not be able to give himself leukemia. Even if he's willing to sit next to an atomic reactor, it might take him twenty years to develop symptoms. So he must rely on people who already have the disease."

Caplan agrees with Veatch that a volunteer army of research subjects "wouldn't wash scientifically." But he does see room for each of us to volunteer for a short while as part of our civic duty—or be called to do so, the way we're called to serve on juries.

"I'm not sure anyone knows what the individual owes the state in terms of medical experimentation," Caplan concluded. "But if medicine becomes publicly funded, through national health insurance, that question may be of great importance."

THE AGENT ORANGE MYSTERY

By Pamela Weintraub

Bill Singley shivered as he trudged past the ramshackle brownstones of South Broad Street. The hefty martial arts instructor made his way to the first-floor office of number 1427 and fell painfully into a chair. Every muscle depleted, each joint throbbing with Philadelphia's latest chill, he wondered whether he'd ever teach karate again.

The young internist who finally invited Singley into the bare inner office didn't look as if he could offer much hope. He simply fixed his patient with a blunt gaze and solemnly began his exam. After 30 minutes Dr. Ronald Codario could tell Singley only that his liver was bloated and his nervous system damaged.

By June 1981, Dr. Codario had Singley hospitalized for a "workup." A body scan and biopsy told him that the distraught patient's scarred liver had deteriorated like an alcoholic's, though

Singley insisted he rarely drank. Then, in the following weeks, Singley's symptoms mounted: His fingers and toes grew numb; his head and abdomen throbbed; he became anxious and confused.

Codario couldn't decipher the cause of the strange illness, but he did know that Singley was a Vietnam veteran. Before long, he started wondering whether the symptoms might not be due to the notorious agent orange — a herbicide that had been dumped on Vietnam to destroy crops that fed and camouflaged enemy troops. Codario told Singley he'd probably been exposed to some kind of toxin and advised him to see a lawyer.

A few weeks later Codario received a call from Hy Mayerson, a Philadelphia attorney who represented vets with illnesses they claimed were caused by agent orange. "Would you like to see some other veterans who've had exposure?" Mayerson asked. "You might be able to help." Codario said sure, and the next day he received weeks of background reading in the mail.

Agent orange, Codario learned, was one of many herbicides sprayed in Vietnam during the 1960s and 1970s. Given its name because it was shipped in orange-striped barrels, agent orange was made largely of a chemical called phenoxyacetic acid. It was usually contaminated with a small molecule known as dioxin, said by some to be the most potent toxin on Earth. Eleven thousand veterans were suing agent orange manufacturers for what they claimed were dioxin's dire side effects: depression, loss of sex drive, joint pain, even cancer. Large numbers of their children, they charged, were being born with deformed hearts, spines, and limbs.

But the experts said there was no real evidence—no *biochemical* evidence—to support such claims. The veterans' troubles, these experts said, were nothing more than a potpourri of unrelated symptoms afflicting the general population in roughly the same proportions.

After examining about 50 or 60 veterans referred by Mayerson, however, Codario observed a strange pattern that made him think otherwise. Like Singley, veteran after veteran complained of personality changes, numbness, aching joints, and extreme sensitivity to sunlight. Amazingly, almost all of them seemed to be describing porphyria (pore-fear-ia), the rare disease that drove King George III mad during the American Revolution.

If Codario could *prove* that his patients had some form of porphyria, he would be the first researcher to establish a biochemical link between agent orange and the veterans' symptoms. With such evidence in hand, he'd be well on his way to helping them get the economic and medical aid they'd been denied for years. With a bit of probing, he might even find a cure.

Classical porphyria, Codario knew, results when the liver churns out massive quantities of chemicals known as porphyrins (pore-fur-ins). Porphyrins produced by healthy livers normally combine with iron and protein to form hemoglobin, the crucial pigment in the red blood cell. But sometimes—because of a genetic deficiency, or because of an unwanted chemical—the liver becomes diseased, manufacturing porphyrins in excess. The extra molecules then travel through the body—to the skin, where they cause huge blisters; to the stomach, where they cause abdominal pain; and to the central nervous system and brain, where they cause numbness, paralysis, and schizophrenia.

Delving into the literature on porphyria, Codario soon found a paper that implied his hunch about agent orange might be correct. The dioxin that contaminated agent orange, the paper suggested , could slip into the nucleus of a living cell and alter genetic material so that the cell produced huge quantities of porphyrin.

By now Codario knew he was hot on the trail of something and began scouring the country for a place that could analyze the veterans' urine for any sign of the disease. Finally he learned of the Watson Laboratory, an internationally acclaimed porphyrin center at Abbott-Northwestern Hospital, in Minneapolis, He placed a call to Zbyslaw J. Petryka, the lab's chief research chemist, and explained his hypothesis. "It's a distinct possibility," Petryka told Codario and volunteered to analyze the veterans' urin himself.

Codario spent the next few weeks collecting urine samples for Petryka. Working late into the night with a group of Philadelphia veterans, he first painted 100 containers pitch-black, since light destroys porphyrins. Then he filled each container with the urine of an ailing patient and got the samples to Petryka by early October.

To test for excess porphyrins in the urine, Petryka used a technique called liquid chromatography: First he poured each urine sample on top of a glass column filled with silica powder, then he waited. Heavier molecules would pass through the powder more quickly than lighter ones; if Petryka knew the weight of a molecule, he could determine its exact identity merely by noting when it reached bottom.

Testing sample after sample, the chemist did indeed find large amounts of relatively heavy porphyrins seeping through the power. Analysis revealed that these porphyrins were similar to those found in the urine of people abusing alcohol, barbituates, and antidepressants. When such patients stopped their abuse, their porphyrin level usually returned to normal. But even when the researchers excluded from their study all veterans with drug or alcohol problems, they found that 60 percent of the urine samples had two to five times more of these porphyrins than expected.

The findings suggested that the veterans had a form of porphyria. But to be surer, Petryka ran the urine through a test called the Ehrlich reaction, based on the action of the Ehrlich solution. This clear solution turns purple when exposed to a variety of chemicals, including porphobilinogen, a substance that yields porphyrins.

By this past winter, Petryka had mixed urine samples from 151 veterans in test tubes filled with transparent pools of Ehrlich solution. Ninety percent of the tubes glowed violet in seconds. But try as he might, he could find so sign of any of the chemicals that usually induce the color change. He concluded that the purple coloration was due to an unknown substance. Ninety percent of the

Vietnam veterans examined by Codario, it seemed, had urine rife with a mystery molecule.

Petryka then found elevated porphyrins and the mystery molecule in the urine of a nine-year-old girl whose mother and father had both served in Vietnam. Although the girl had never been in Vietnam herself, she suffered excruciating pain just as the veterans did: She woke up screaming at night because her ribs ached, and she walked on her toes because her feet hurt.

Petryka has spent the last six months searching for the unknown molecule in the veterans' urine, but so far he's had little luck. "Until the molecule is isolated," he cautions, "we cannot begin to say just *how* it has affected the veterans." Indeed, although the evidence indicates that agent orange is linked to severe physiological problems, the researchers must do far more work before they can absolutely prove that the veterans have a disease.

But Codario, nevertheless, feels the veterans cannot wait for all the answers. *Any* form of porphyria, he explains, can worsen from year to year.

To head off the symptoms, Codario hopes for FDA approval to test a drug called hematin, which inhibits the enzymes that spur porphyrin production. He also suggests there may be a way of eliminating the original toxin, the dioxin itself. Studies with animals, he notes, indicate that dioxin tends to stay in the body indefinitely, circulating from the liver through the bile fluid and back to the liver again. But if a chemical could bind to dioxin during the cycle, preventing it from reentering the liver, it might pass out of the body and stop provoking porphyrin production once and for all. Just such a drug, Codario adds, was recently used to bind molecules of kepone, a poisonous pesticide that behaves like dioxin; the same drug, or one like it, might be made to fight dioxin as well.

The ultimate answer may be far more complex. Vietnam veterans were exposed to a mixture of *15* herbicides and pesticides with names ranging from agent blue (arsenic) to agent purple to agent pink. The soldiers absorbed each of these with the air they breathed, the water they drank, and the food they ate. The combined effect may forever be inestimable.

But, as Codario says, "Even if we never solve the mystery completely, the important thing is to stop telling the veterans there's nothing wrong with them. One hundred fifty of the two hundred people I've examined have porphyrin problems, numb fingers and hands, and an unknown molecule coursing through their systems. It's time to quit the denials and help."

THIS WAY OUT

By Roger M. Williams

On a late March morning in 1975, in a country house in England, Derek Humphry handed his wife a lethal potion of sleeping pills and painkillers mixed with coffee. Jean Humphry, forty-two, was dying of bone cancer. She was determined to take her life, with her husband's emotional support and active assistance.

As the Humphrys made their final preparations, Derek marveled at Jean's calmness and attention to detail. When he broke into tears, she reminded him gently, "I can't take any more of this cancer. I'd rather die peacefully today, enjoying your presence and love in my own home, than in some grim hospital after being knocked senseless with drugs for a couple of weeks. This is the best way."

Jean Humphry did die that morning. Derek, a journalist, could have kept the manner of his wife's death private, but he chose to reveal publicly this dark area of human affairs: the treatment of the terminally ill. Humphry published *Jean's Way*, his account of the entire episode, which aroused controversy in Great Britain and far beyond. Questioned by the police, he freely confessed to having "aided and abetted suicide"—a crime in England and much of the United States. The authorities declined to prosecute.

Derek Humphry now lives in Santa Monica, California, where he leads a right-to-die movement—that is, the right of an aged or terminally ill person to will his or her own death, with the understanding, or perhaps even the complicity, of family, friends, and physicians.

The practice is more properly termed voluntary euthanasia. It is being promoted with increasing vigor by organizations in this country and abroad. Hemlock, an aptly named group that Humphry founded a year ago, now numbers about 1,500 members, with the total growing at the rate of 30 a week. Most of the members are couples in the thirty-to-fifty-year age bracket; 10 percent are facing a terminal illness. "We have all types," Humphry says, "including doctors, nurses, and clergymen."

Hemlock has just made available to its membership a controversial book that reports, with sympathy and gritty detail, the true accounts of people who ended or tried to end lives they regarded as no longer livable. Although suicide tips can certainly be gleaned from these stories, Humphry emphasizes that the book concerns life as much as death: "It counsels survival as long as possible and, when it's no longer possible, sensible preparation for the end, that is, dealing with matters of timing, who to tell and not to tell, psychological and legal effects on one's family, and so forth."

Far more explicit—and socially abrasive—is a how-to guide to suicide that Hemlock's British counterpart, Exit, is struggling to publish over fierce opposition. This book-to-be contains recommendations against various methods of suicide along with lucid descriptions of five approaches that really work. Exit, which presently faces litigation in Great Britain, is unwilling to reveal many details. But one method involves intentional drug overdose, with a chart that lists fatal amounts of some 200 prescription and nonprescription drugs. The book also discusses the pros and cons of death by asphyxiation and by electrocution in the bathtub.

"We recommend the reasonably peaceful and nonviolent ways," says Nicholas Reed, Exit's general secretary. "No shooting or hanging. We come out against wrist slashing, because it hardly ever works and makes a mess of the hands, and against common overdoses, such as aspirin and painkillers, which just damage the body." The book boasts an eloquent and moving introduction by the eminent philosopher of science Arthur Koestler, a staunch supporter of Exit.

Derek Humphry predicts that voluntary euthanasia "will be the next major social issue." Demographic studies lend credence to his viewpoint. The American birth rate has been declining steadily since the 1920s, with the exception of the postwar baby boom. If present reproduction trends continue, an estimated one third of the U.S. population will be old in 40 years' time. Dialysis machines, respirators, chemotherapy — these and other medical technologies keep the elderly alive longer with fewer members of the younger generation to care for the sick and the dying. More and more diseases will end in lingering death, at a staggering financial cost to survivors or, through medical insurance, to the public at large. How many of us would opt for a pain-free and dignified way out of such predicaments to help save our families?

The right-to-die movement is gaining on numerous fronts. The dissemination of millions of so-called living wills is perhaps the most tangible sign of its enormous following. These wills direct medical authorities not to prolong life if the signer has become terminally ill. They were first accorded legal status in 1976, when California passed a Natural Death Act, which gives competent adults the power to discontinue life-sustaining treatment. Under the law, any doctor who feels his ethical principles violated can remove himself from a case rather than be a party to euthanasia.

Besides California, the following states now have natural-death legislation on the books: Arkansas, Idaho, Kansas, Nevada, New Mexico, North Carolina, Oregon, Texas, and Washington. Movement activists consider the laws of Kansas, New Mexico, and Washington the best in that they permit the necessary document to be drawn up at any time, not just when an individual becomes terminally ill.

"That's very important," says Alice V. Mehling, of the Society for the Right to Die (SRD), one of two long-established groups working to legalize such wills. "A dying patient may not be *able* to make his wishes known. This statement should be treated like the last will and testament; what if the law said you could execute a will only when you're terminal?"

SRD now has right-to-die committees in several states. The committees lobby for natural-death acts and keep the public informed of developments favorable to the cause. A second organization, Concern for Dying (CFD), split from SRD several years ago and now concentrates on what it calls educational activities, including information on living wills. A. J. Levenson, executive director of CFD, says, "We believe legislation is unnecessary, except perhaps to protect the doctor involved against criminal charges. Actually, we're not certain doctors *should* be protected with a blanket release. They should be held accountable for the practice of sound medicine."

As an organized cause in the United States, voluntary euthanasia dates from 1937. In England it dates from two years earlier, and it is England's Exit that led the way into an uncharted part of right-to-die territory—the dissemination of self help suicide information. Exit succeeded the original Voluntary Euthanasia Society, which had been known for its British reserve and strong antipathy toward suicide.

Bearded young Nicholas Reed changed all

that. He marketed euthanasia aggressively and made the society at least neutral on the issue of suicide. Yet Reed had to wage a three-year internal struggle to get Exit's executive committee to agree to publish the suicide handbook, *A Guide to Self-Deliverance*.

When news of the tempest hit the press early last year, interest in both the handbook and the Exit organization soared. In less than nine months membership quadrupled, reaching 8,000. Not counting the British, Exit's home constituents, Americans account for twice as many respondents as any other nationality. By June 1980 the group had enlisted 250 American members, receiving an average of ten queries a day from the United States. (The enrollment categories, with a touch of black humor, include "life member.")

A basketful of recent letters to Exit produced at least a dozen bearing Stateside addresses:

A California woman: "My religion does not condone suicide; however, my parents are in their eighties, and I had cancer in 1976. Should it reoccur, I want to make a decision for myself, and to be supportive of my parents, regarding a dignified death."

A California man: "I'm over sixty years old, rather ill, and, if at all possible, I [underscored three times] want to make a decision for deliverance."

A Providence, Rhode Island, man: "Having been brought up under strict Roman Catholic tradition. I appreciate hearing that there are those who do not believe one must suffer the agonies of terminal illnesses that fate deals."

An Ohio woman, a "cancer patient": "I consider myself very sane. . . . I want very much to live if at all possible, but I do not wish to be a useless vegetable or a financial and emotional problem."

Among other Americans who have requested either information or the suicide handbook itself were a chiropractor from New Jersey and the coordinator of Late Life Counseling Services at a large Midwestern medical center.

This correspondence is received, with sympathy approaching passion, by the Exit staff members, almost all of whom have been personally touched by death. One elderly woman, a former actress who did not want to be identified, told me of watching her father succumb to cancer: "They said he'd last six months, but he dragged on for sixteen. In the middle of that, he had a heart attack, and the doctors brought him 'round—to die of cancer. Right now I have a very good friend with multiple sclerosis. She'll soon be bedridden and in a bad way. I definitely feel that euthanasia is the answer for her, and so does she."

Janet Burnell, also of Exit, says it has "been my fate" to see a succession of friends die lingering and painful deaths. "Most people who condemn euthanasia," she observes, "have never been asked by someone close to help them die."

Marsh Dickson, a sprightly seventy-two-year-old, saw his mother, who had a brain tumor, botch a suicide attempt with an underdose of pills and his wife, suffering with multiple sclerosis, die after a wholly debilitating slide.

But Dickson's most vivid memory is of a Burmese jungle trail in World War II. When his British Army unit was ambushed there by Japanese soldiers and one of his men was "hoplessly" wounded, Dickson says, "I did what the man begged me to do — put him out of his misery with a bullet. If my own wife had asked, I'd have done exactly the same for her."

Experiences like those are what prompted Exit to publish *A Guide to Self-Deliverance*, thereby raising the ethical dilemma of suicide for all ages, rather than simply the question of euthanasia for the elderly. Although half of the handbook is devoted, in Reed's words, to "why *not* to commit suicide," the other half, which details the five deadly ways, has provoked alarm and condemnation.

At this writing, publication was still being delayed for fear of prosecution. Meanwhile Exit's Scottish offshoot, not bound by English law, has already published a version of the book, entitled *How to Die with Dignity*. And one, Dutch euthanasia society, stimulated by Exit's efforts, has put out a slim, technical volume instructing physicians on dosages and other procedures that will ensure the success of "justified euthanasia."

Even without its handbook, English Exit has got into trouble with the law. Last summer London police summoned Reed for questioning about the suicide of Mrs. Hettie Crystal, a multiple sclerosis patient who had been in touch with Exit shortly before her death in December 1979. A few months later Reed and Exit volunteer worker Mark Lyons were charged in connection with aiding and abetting in Mrs. Crystal's death. Neither Reed nor Lyons has yet pleaded to the charges, but the Exit organization intends to support them fully in court.

Exit's campaign has not gone unchallenged. The British Medical Association and the Samaritans, an English-based group that "befriends the deeply troubled," have issued statements questioning euthanasia and condemning the handbook. Samaritans official Jean Burt rests her case on studies of persons who attempted suicide and failed: "Eighty percent were glad to be still alive." She further points out that a suicide attempt may not be meant to end in death, but may be a cry for help. Ms. Burt deplores making an Exit-style handbook available to teen-agers, "whose moods go up and down like yo-yos."

Those objections were put to Sheila Little, seventy-four, who fields tough questions on Exit's behalf. The next decade will see an increase of 43 percent in the number of Britons over eighty-five, Miss Little declared, "but there will not be a parallel increase in the number of caring relatives or facilities looking after them." Increasing numbers of the elderly will therefore prefer to die, and they should be allowed to do so.

As for the handbook, Miss Little emphasizes that it will be available only to members of at least three months' standing. That, she said, will mitigate the problem of having copies fall into the hands of persons who are unstable or temporarily depressed. But what if the handbook is passed around or Xeroxed? "Our members are responsible people, and we will include in the mailing a very firm statement about how they should keep the material under cover. However, if somebody *steals* a handbook or if a given member turns out not to be very honest, Exit can hardly be held responsible."

Pressed on that point, Miss Little added, "There will certainly be one or two unfortunate incidents. But you need to weigh those against the welfare of six thousand or seven thousand elderly people [in Great Britain], lying in pain and suffering a needless prolongation of the dying process."

Let Me Die Before I Wake, Hemlock's version of the handbook, will be "more human, more loving" than Exit's, Humphry says. "It will not be a how-to guide but a compilation of people's acts of voluntary euthanasia, told in their words. As such, our lawyers assure us, it will have First Amendment protection." Hemlock, like Exit, will sell handbooks only to members of three months' standing.

Both CFD and SRD decided not to publish anything resembling Exit's handbook. "Our decision was unanimous and based on two factors," says Mrs. Levenson, of CFD. "First, terminating one's life is the most drastic step a person can take, and anything that makes it easier is probably not good. Second, promoting the acceptability of suicide could have a rebound effect on the elderly, with old people telling themselves, 'I have no right to be alive and sick and a burden on others. I have a duty to kill myself.' The United States has done a terrible job of caring for its elderly. We don't favor anything that relieves society of its responsibility for improving their lot."

Humphry readily agrees. Asked whether he thinks that proeuthanasia material should be distributed among the aged, he replies, "Definitely not. I don't favor even making them aware of the option, because that would imply an obligation on their part to consider it." Hemlock, he adds, is careful not to proselytize. "People must hear of us in one way or another and come join. Morally and legally, we feel, that's the necessary approach. It's all right to talk in general terms about voluntary euthanasia or 'assisted suicide.' But it's not all right to say to a person, 'I think you should die. Take forty Seconals.' "

SFD, meanwhile, intends to press nationwide for natural-death legislation. Alice Mehling says that the group has encountered two principal objections on the legislative level. "One is that a natural-death law will open the door to mercy killing, and the other is that there's no need for such a law, because doctors are already permitting or practicing voluntary euthanasia." Mrs. Mehling insists that the record since passage of the first act shows no trend toward mercy killing. "There hasn't been a bit of litigation under any of the laws, and the question of abuse hasn't been seriously raised. As for the laws' being unnecessary, not all hospitals are going to honor a living will without legislation behind them. Besides, once a person is connected to a [life-sustaining] machine, it's difficult to have the treatment stopped."

Where will it all lead? To indiscriminate, needless suicide? To that and worse, says Malcolm

Muggeridge, the English social critic and curmudgeon-at-large. Exit, Muggeridge says, "represents the trend toward total paganism, toward regarding human beings as merely bodies, *animal* bodies. If that's all they are, you don't worry about putting them to death. But if you believe men are created by God and have souls, such a choice would not arise."

Muggeridge excoriates Exit's suicide handbook as "completely the devil's work. If a man consciously and sincerely wants to die, all right. I think he's committing a sin, but people do sin, as we know. In any case, experience shows that people think favorably about euthanasia for themselves when they're well. When they become ill and are actually confronted with death, they wish to remain alive."

Right-to-die advocates dismiss arguments framed in the Muggeridge manner as at best unrealistic. Acceptance of voluntary euthanasia, they say, will bring a dramatic reduction in unnecessary suffering among the dying, as well as a new and healthy respect for a human being's control over his own life. "Eighty percent of us are going to die in hospitals," Mrs. Mehling says. "None of us know under what circimstances, but we do know that the concept of individual decision making is really gaining greater acceptance."

At least one prominent psychiatrist, the renegade Dr. Thomas Szasz, argues that none of the present right-to-die advocates are going nearly far enough. Dr. Szasz, who believes that "although suicide is not necessarily good, it's your right," insists that not only information on lethal drugs but the drugs themselves should be made generally available. He dismisses concern over euthanasia. Suicide is the issue, he says, and it has been given a bum rap: "Suicide bears the same relation to murder as masturbation does to rape. It's nobody's business but that of the person who does it. Yet we link *sui*cide and *homi*cide, instead of using a sensible term like *self-determined death.*"

Few of us, including leading proponents of the right to die, would go all the way with Thomas Szasz. But it is hard to dispute his contention that the issue raises "one of the fundamental questions of the contemporary social world."

MORE THRILLING READING!

THE LUCIFER DIRECTIVE   (1353, $3.50)
by Jon Land
Terrorists are outgunning agents, and events are outracing governments. It's all part of a sequence of destruction shrouded in mystery. And the only ones who hold key pieces of the bloody puzzle are a New England college student and an old Israeli freedom fighter. From opposite ends of the globe, they must somehow stop the final fatal command!

THE DOOMSDAY SPIRAL   (1175, $2.95)
by Jon Land
Alabaster—master assassin and sometimes Mossad agent—races against time and operatives from every major service in order to control and kill a genetic nightmare let loose in America. Death awaits around each corner as the tension mounts and doomsday comes ever closer!

DEPTH FORCE   (1355, $2.95)
by Irving A. Greenfield
Built in secrecy, launched in silence, and manned by a phantom crew, *The Shark* is America's unique high technology submarine whose mission is to stop the Soviets from dominating the seas. As far as the U.S. government is concerned, *The Shark* doesn't exist. Its orders are explicit: if in danger of capture, self-destruct! So the only way to stay alive is to dive deep and strike hard!